Dietmar Ferger

Fountain of Youth Water

From the Normal to the Healthy with ionised water

Understanding and using alkaline and acidic ionised water

FOUNTAIN OF YOUTH WATER

From the Normal to the Healthy
with ionised water

Understanding and using
alkaline and acidic ionised water

A comprehensive guide to the
understanding of water
and to health and well-being by

Dietmar Ferger

Dietmar Ferger

Fountain of Youth Water – from the Normal to the Healthy with ionised water

Understanding and using alkaline and acidic ionised water

© 2022 Dietmar Ferger

1st English edition 2022

Ingram Spark Edition 2022

ISBN print edition: 978-3-910637-00-9

ISBN E-Book: 978-3-910637-01-6

Also available as KDP Edition via Amazon with the ISBN 979-8-62285014-1

For more information, including an up-to-date overview of studies, reviews and reports on the effects of ionised water, please visit **www.fountain-of-youth-water.com**.

First published in 2002 in German, now in the 7th updated edition

    Original German title:

    Jungbrunnenwasser – vom Normalen zum Gesunden mit ionisiertem Wasser

    Basisches Aktivwasser und saures Oxidwasser verstehen und anwenden

    7th German edition, 2002 – 2023

    Print version: ISBN: 978-3-9810897-5-2

    E-Book: ISBN: 978-3-9810897-9-0

Design, graphics and translation: Dietmar Ferger

Fonts: Title: Ubuntu

    Content: Clear Sans

This book is written in British English

Content

About the author

Dietmar Ferger is graduate engineer in environmental protection and water technology, preventive care specialist and teacher. Since many years his main interest is the interrelation between water and health, his work focuses on health, detoxification and holistic concepts of health prevention. Furthermore, he is member of the Presidium of the German Naturopathy Society, the oldest organisation of this kind in Europe.

Besides of lectures at congresses and publications in professional and popular magazines, he has published various books like

• "Der Weg zurück in die Jugend" (Translation of the book "Reverse Aging" by Sang Whang)

• "Pneumobalance" (translation from Russian, by Dr Sergei Zinatulin

• "Sonnenkind Michelle" (Translation of "A gift called Michelle" by Barbara Desrochers)

Contact: **www.fountain-of-youth-water.com**

Preface by Professor Maximilian Gege

"Without water, there is no salvation" has been said by Goethe – and he is right:

Water is our elixir of life, carrying out many vital tasks in our body. While we can survive without solid food for several weeks, we can only spare water for a maximum of two to four days.

Therefore, there are three perspectives from which to look at water: taste, health effect and the ecological and social framework conditions. Since 2010, we drink alkaline ionised water in the "Haus der Zukunft" ("House of Future"). It convinces us in all three aspects mentioned above:

- It tastes significantly better than the untreated Hamburg tap water; tea or coffee prepared with this water have a more intense flavour.

- Convincing are the health aspects too. 10% of Germanys gross national product is spent on the treatment of illnesses, the number of sick people increases and thus also the economic damage caused by loss of work and earnings. This is an alarming signal. Any convincing approach to reduce this continuously rising quota in a side-effect-free, economically viable and affordable way must be intensively promoted and supported and subjected to an unprejudiced test. In addition, alkaline ionised water entices you to drink more – an important positive health effect in the hectic rush of the office day – and also to promote alertness, balance and well-being.

- From the ecological point of view, alkaline ionised water is far superior to all purchased alternatives offered by the mineral water industry. In 2009, Germans consumed around 130 litres of bottled water or 15 to 20 mineral water crates per capita. Every year, a family of five tows up to 100 crates into the apartment, which were previously driven by truck from the bottling plant over hundreds of kilometres to the beverage- or supermarket. These are, for example, 1'000 plastic bottles of 1 litre each, which, when placed one behind the other, make up a distance of 300 meters. More than 10% of this water still comes from abroad, with a particularly long "journey". The international mineral waters travel an average of around 850 kilometres until they quench our thirst.

Alkaline ionised water combines taste and health improvement with ecological reason and sustainability. I gave away this book to many friends and hope that it finds many more readers. It helps to increase knowledge about water in general, the role of water in our human body and its health significance.

Professor Maximilian Gege, 2011
Chairman of „Bundesdeutschen Arbeitskreis für Umweltbewusstes Management (B.A.U.M.) e.V.,
(All-German Working Group for Environmentally Friendly Management), Hamburg

Preface by the author for the first English edition

Some English-speaking friends convinced me to translate my book „Jungbrunnenwasser", which has been sold in its German version up to now in nearly 20.000 copies and is now in its seventh edition.

Water is a fascinating element. Researching this topic for many years, I have met scientists who have been intensively involved with water for decades – and are still at the beginning of their research. **Therefore, a book about water can only be a provisional appraisal and represent the current state of knowledge.**

This book is about "ionised water", a machine-made, functional water with properties that are very useful for nature and mankind.

Albert Szent-Gyorgyi M.D., the Nobel laureate and discoverer of Vitamin C, wrote that *"ageing symptoms ... are always associated with a slow shrivelling of our living tissue, accompanied by damage caused by reactive oxygen species (ROS)"* - we know today that alkaline ionised water permanently hydrates the body tissues and neutralizes ROS with gaseous hydrogen. So, it is certainly not presumptuous to call it "**Fountain of Youth Water**" ... Soviet scientists who researched it before Perestroika even called it "**The Water of Life**".

The ionisation of water is a "treatment" of water with technical or natural electric energy, being among the most significant developments in the diverse "water markets" since the development of reverse osmosis technology. It is interesting to note that the intense Soviet Russian research on ionised water was simply stopped after the collapse of the Soviet Union, and that the development in Japan and Korea led to technical perfection over decades without anyone in the West noticing. Except for a few lectures by Japanese scientists at international congresses, for a long time there were no scientific sources that were accessible without Japanese or Korean language skills.

In 1990, the book "**Reverse Aging**" opened the "Gate of Knowledge" for the English-speaking world. The author *Sang Whang (†)*, an American engineer of Korean descent, was able to evaluate the original sources and embed them in a Western scientific context. I translated it into German and published it in 2002.

Since understanding the book "Reverse Aging", I see it as my task to inform scientists, politicians, therapists and consumers about alkaline ionised water and its positive potential for the rehabilitation of our prohibitively expensive public health, for the prevention of increasing lifestyle and geriatric diseases and for the optimization of human health and zest for life.

Since 2003, we are drinking alkaline ionised water and, since 2016, hydrogen water. Our kids never wanted to drink Coke or other soft drinks and hardly needed any sick-leave from school.

Other users report success in the development of their health and performance, like cellulite disappearing within 4 weeks, bedridden patients becoming active again, high blood pressure or intraocular pressure going down, and far more.

Mainly Japanese studies have shown that alkaline ionised water and hydrogen water are not only simple and effective methods of prevention – if prevention is not only understood as a series of more or less meaningful vaccinations or preventive screenings for early detection of diseases –, but also supportive in the treatment of lifestyle and geriatric diseases.

Although alkaline ionised water and hydrogen water can be effective, simple and cost-effective means of health care and enhancing quality of life and performance, they are not (yet) recognized in the "western" medicine, as no studies accepted by the rules of the western scientific community have been carried out. It is therefore important to stress that the findings cited in this book are based on own or third-party observations, reports and conclusions, but not on studies recognized in "western" science.

Therefore, this book is not intended to replace a doctor or therapist who should always be consulted on acute or chronic conditions.

The ignorance of western science and society also has far-reaching consequences for nature and the environment, because the use of anolyte and catholyte in agriculture and animal breeding and also the use of anolyte as a highly effective and side-effect free disinfectant in hospitals and – as in the fight against the corona virus in China – in fighting epidemics would avoid the use of antibiotics and chemical disinfectants, which in the long term and persistently contaminate water, soil and the environment.

With this in mind, I wish you an interesting read with the request that you pass on or recommend this book to people who are interested in holistic health and preserving the environment. It is not without reason that most of the Korean and Japanese households nowadays are equipped with a water ioniser or another similar device for treating and enhancing their drinking water.

Dietmar Ferger
environmental engineer and preventologist

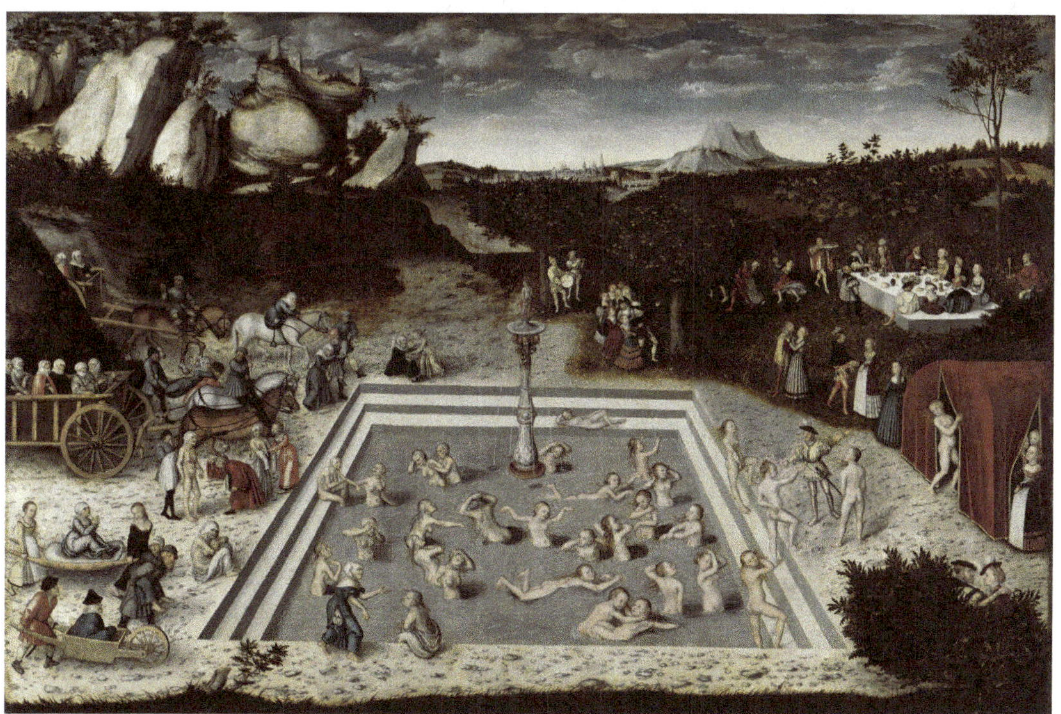

Fountain of youth, painting by Lucas Cranach the Elder from the year 1546
(Source: Wikimedia)

The fairy tale of the Fountain of Youth Water

Mankind dreams of the „Fountain of Youth" since ancient times. It is a dream of the „Water of Life", washing away age and diseases, sung about in many fairy tales and legends and can be found in medieval portrayals.

Today, we do not take fairy tales literally anymore and have stopped searching for the proverbial „Fountain of Youth", like the medieval alchemists. Nevertheless, those fairy tales still contain much more than just a spark of truth, since realizing that water is more than just H_2O pervades the evolution of mankind.

Even though today the rational natural sciences, the pharmaceutical industry and the purely materialistic, mechanical world view dominate the universities and the official science, there are many excellent scientists and researchers exploring the structures of water, treating and enhancing water with holistic methods, giving it properties that are beyond the understanding of materialistic thinking. In the past, they were often condemned and burned as heretics or witches, today they are outsiders in the science business.

For laymen it is often very difficult to evaluate and understand the properties of "miraculous waters", since the threshold between deep knowledge and unscrupulous money-making is rather narrow. Only with extended horizons in physics and biology, like the so-called quantum physics or quantum biology, one can attempt to understand and to explain the properties of these miraculous waters and their scientific background.

The ignorance of conventional science about the secrets of water is the reason why technologies developed with this ignorance have a destructive effect on water. What harms water also harms nature and man, what is beneficial to water is also beneficial to nature and man, a "water-loving" technology is always a natural and humane technology.

For example, the global network of high-voltage power lines with hundreds of thousands of volts affects the electric properties of the groundwater and destroys its natural balance and thus any potential healing effect – it reaches even the most remote spring that originates from the groundwater. The multiple microwave radiations in the atmosphere, caused by radar, cell phones and other wireless transmissions, affect every water molecule in the falling raindrop, every snowflake, so that all information of the cosmos brought down by this water molecules is erased or mutilated. The water coming out of our pipes is mixed with chemicals in the water-works, pressed, squeezed and forced to flow straight and untwisted, usually even parallel to power lines and data cables, which destroy its structures even further.

Chapter 1: Water, the Chemistry of Life

If we want to determine whether there is life – as we imagine life to be – on Mars or other planets, scientists are looking for traces of water first. Why water is so important? Life on earth depends on water, in water, life had its origin. Depending on their habitat, the body of living beings consists of 70 to 95% of water. In plants and animals, all chemical reactions supporting life take place with the help of water. Thereby, water not only provides the medium in which the reactions take place, but water is often also an important component of these reactions.

The Structure of Atoms

In order to understand the water phenomenon, we have to enter the world of atoms (from Greek atomos = indivisible), the smallest particles. One may imagine these atoms being structured like our solar system: negatively charged particles, the electrons, circle around the nucleus, consisting of protons, positively charged particles, and neutrons, particles without charge. They circle in different layers, the so-called "shells". As with the planets, there are several distances from the nucleus, at which the electrons move. Unlike the planets, however, it is not possible to calculate the location of an electron on his assigned shell, so physicists speak of a so-called "probability density", which means the probability that the electron is exactly where it is supposed to be.

The first shell consists of a maximum of two, the second and third shell of a maximum of eight electrons. Each atom has the desire to complete its outermost shell by filling it with the maximum number of electrons. Only the electrons of the respective outermost shell, the **valence electrons**, are significant for a chemical reaction, they determine the character of the atom.

Furthermore, electrons always "want" to be in pairs. A **paired electron** is therefore less reactive than a so-called **unpaired** electron.

Even if, in order to make things easier to understand, the electron orbits are always drawn in concentric circles around the atomic nucleus, the actual proportions correspond roughly to those in our solar system:: Imagine the atomic nucleus of protons and neutrons as a ping-pong ball located in the middle of a huge stadium, about as heavy as the entire stadium, the innermost ring of electrons revolves approximately at the distance of the farthest rows of seats and is about the size of a pinhead, which can be found anywhere and nowhere at this distance. The next electron orbit around the ping-pong ball in the middle of the stadium may be as far away as the stadium's parking lot or the helicopter above it, from which the game is filmed. The "quantum space" between the electron orbits and the atomic nucleus is filled by an energy field of interactions between electrons and atomic nucleus.

According to the current state of research, the protons and neutrons that make up the "ping-pong ball" in the stadium consist of the smallest particles, the so-called quarks, which in turn consist of three "vortexes", which are – according to the superstring theory – one-dimensional and without any mass. These vortexes – and thus also the character of the matter – can be influenced: Research by the Russian-American physicist *Yuri Kronn* and others suggests that the character of the energy vortexes and thus also of matter can be changed by building up mental energy fields – especially in water and in all living matter containing water.

This short and, of course, incomplete journey into quantum physics is intended to broaden the understanding of matter in general and of water and in particular, an understanding mainly influenced by our senses of sight and touch. This can make homeopathy and other energetic phenomena become conceivable.

The number of protons and neutrons in the nucleus characterizes an atom and assigns it its place in the periodic table of the elements – each element of the periodic table is uniquely determined by the number of protons and neutrons in the nucleus. In the case of a single, non-electrically charged atom, there is a numerical equilibrium between protons in the nucleus and electrons in the orbits. If electrons are removed from the orbit or if new electrons are added, the atom is called **positively or negatively "ionised"** - the number of protons always remains the same and can only be changed by nuclear fission, which produces another element.

The Water Molecule

A water molecule with the chemical formula H_2O contains two atoms of hydrogen and one atom of oxygen. The water molecule has the shape of a tetrahedron, i.e. an equilateral pyramid with a triangular base.

The hydrogen atom consists of a proton in the atomic nucleus and an electron in the atomic shell. Hydrogen ionises rapidly by losing its single electron and thus becomes a positively charged H^+, an isolated proton, because hydrogen atom has no neutrons.

The oxygen atom consists of eight protons plus eight neutrons in the nucleus and eight electrons, of which two are on the inner shell and thus are ineffective for the chemical reaction. Thus, oxygen has six valence electrons, two of which are unpaired. If it now combines with two hydrogen atoms, it receives a share of the two hydrogen electrons and both unpaired oxygen electrons receive a partner electron. The water molecule thus formed has a total of eight paired valence electrons on the outer shell - the oxygen has fulfilled its "desire" for eight electrons on the second shell, sharing the two electrons of the hydrogen atoms in so-called "**covalent bonds**". The resulting electromagnetic attraction forces create special positions of the electrons and an asymmetric molecule, in which hydrogen atoms form an angle of 104.5 ° with oxygen (instead of mathematically calculated 109.5 °).

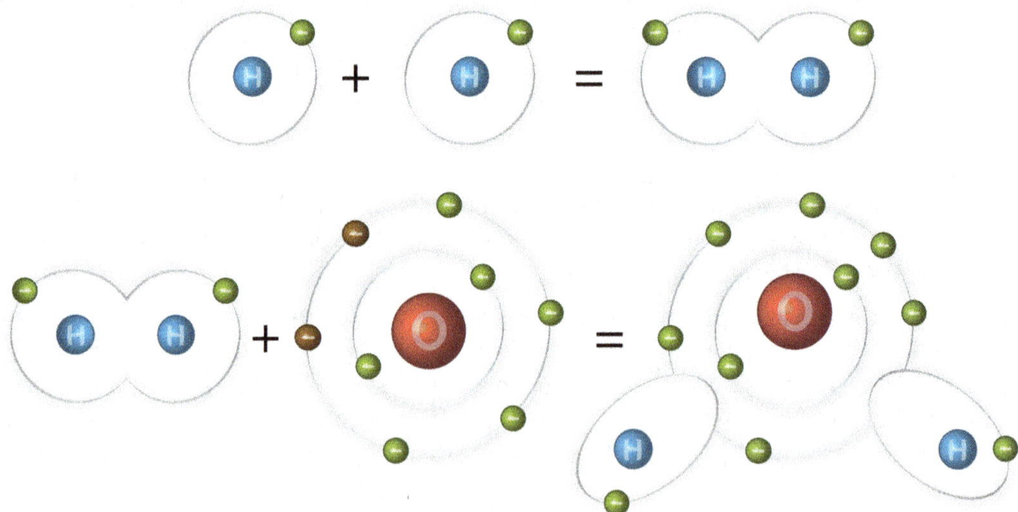

Fig. 1 (top): Hydrogen H always occurs in nature as hydrogen molecule H_2

Fig. 2 (bottom): A hydrogen molecule H_2 and an oxygen atom O form a water molecule H_2O. The two unpaired electrons are red.

The polarity of the water molecule is crucial!

As the three atoms in a water molecule have different sizes - the oxygen atom is much larger than the two hydrogen atoms -, the electrons are attracted to different degrees by the respective atomic nuclei. The attraction of an atom for electrons is called "**electronegativity**". With a value of 3.5, the electronegativity of oxygen is almost twice as large as that of hydrogen with 2.1. This has considerable impact on the electrons of the two hydrogen atoms: these common electrons "binding" together the water molecule is pulled closer to the oxygen, resulting in a negative partial charge (δ^-) at the opposite end of the molecule; whereas the two hydrogen atoms have less electrons and thus a positive partial charge occurs there (δ^+).

Molecules which – like a magnet – have opposite charged ends are called dipoles. Since the difference in electronegativity of water molecules is very high, water is a strong dipole. This polarity makes water a universal and strong solvent. Due to its strong polarity, it is able to dissolve all polar substances and to build hydrogen bonds, which are primarily accountable for the special geometry and thus for the reaction of proteins and nucleic acids.

This positive and negative charge causes water to also react to external magnetic influences – a property that enables magnetic treatment of limestone-rich water, for example.

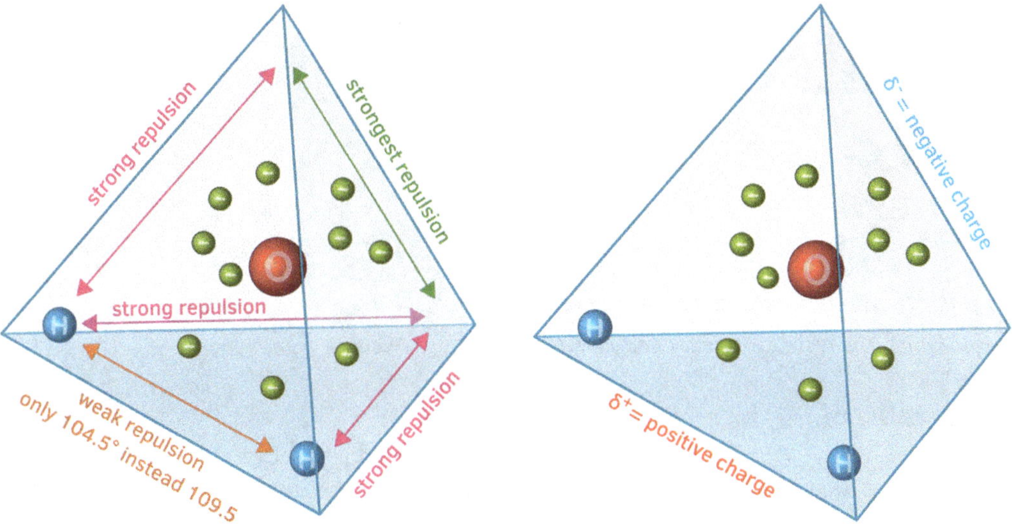

Fig. 3 (left): The geometry of a water molecule

Fig. 4 (right): The unequal distribution of electrons shows the dipole character of a water molecule

Hydrogen bonds enable our life

Water molecules form intermolecular bonds to adjacent water molecules by attraction forces between the negative end of a molecule and the positive end of the adjacent molecule. This is comparable to the attraction of one magnet to another magnet. Thus, forms of "stacked" tetrahedrons of water molecules are formed in space.

The so-called **hydrogen bonds** are only a fraction as strong as the binding forces within a molecule. Therefore, they can be very easily built up and also broken down again. These weak compounds play a crucial role in the stabilization of many large organic molecules. Being so weak, they can be quickly broken down and rebuilt in biological and physiological reactions. **This disintegration and renewal enable the chemistry of life.**

Hydrogen bonds are also causing the surface tension of water (the formation of water drops, "skin of the water") and its relatively high boiling point of 100°C / 212°F – analogous to other substances and according to the laws of chemistry and physics, water should actually be gaseous at room temperature, have a melting point of -120°C / -148°F and a boiling point of -75°C / -103°F. The hydrogen bonds also cause water to have its highest density at 4°C / 39°F: Below this temperature, ice crystals are formed that enclose hollow spaces and require more volume – which is why ice floats on water. Above this temperature, water molecules are stimulated to vibrate and also require more volume. Hydrogen bonds are thus causing most of the so-called **63 "anomalies" of water** known so far, which make life on earth possible.

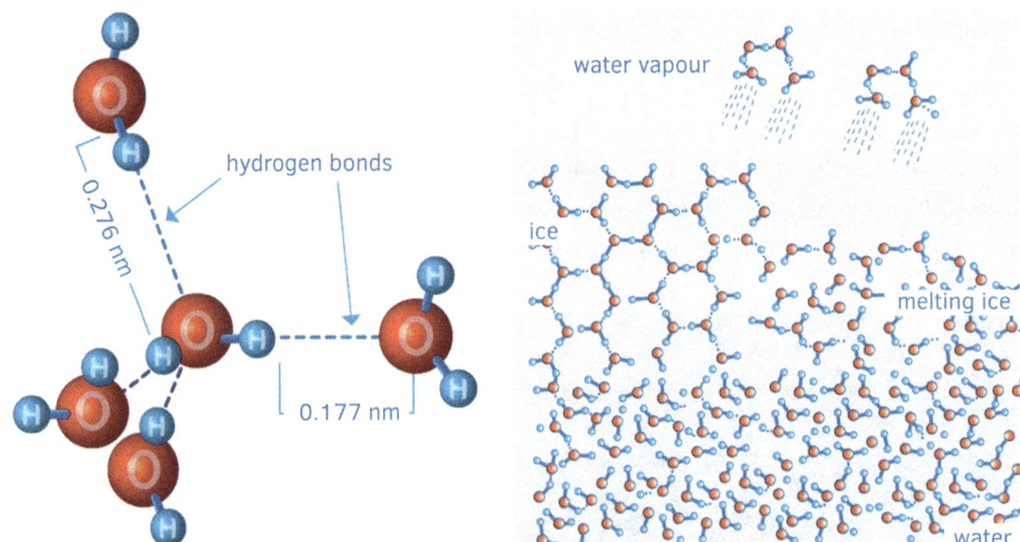

Fig. 5 (left): Hydrogen bonding between several water molecules

Fig. 6 (right): The state forms of water: liquid water – ice - steam

Water cluster

Several water molecules jointly form "**water clusters**", held together by hydrogen bonds. These are structures whose properties are still being researched. A model for understanding water clusters says, that the water molecules exchange their bonds mainly within this water clusters and that thus a certain number of molecules form a more or less large cluster, appearing outwardly as one single unit and reacting with other molecules only on its surface.

Another model says, that an ideal water cluster has the geometric shape like an icosahedron, a 20-faced polyhedron, composed of tetrahedrons. Like the tetrahedron, the icosahedron is one of the so-called five "Platonic solids". Twenty tetrahedrons can nearly form one icosahedron, not exactly, but leaving a "living space", a remainder, a gap. Just as the water molecule does not form an exact tetrahedron, but leaves some "space for living", according to this model the water cluster is not an exact icosahedron, but rather a spatial structure composed of – likewise not exact – tetrahedron-like space formations, similar to an icosahedron.

The Platonic solids already played an important role in Greek science and philosophy. In Plato's Academy, they were considered as representatives of the five elements:

- Fire: tetrahedron
- Water: icosahedron

- Air: octahedron
- Earth: cube
- Ether: Dodecahedron

Thus, in Greek science, the icosahedron was also assigned to water – perhaps also influenced by the observation of ice or snow crystals, in which the icosahedral structure become visible

Although they are held together only by weak hydrogen bonds, these water clusters are so stable that under normal pressure conditions, isolated water molecules only appear at temperatures above about 375°C / 707°F, or at extremely low pressure, like in the uppermost layers of the atmosphere.

The special structure of the hydrogen bonds, the electrical voltage between the hydrogen and the oxygen side present in the water molecule dipole, the possibility that ionised hydrogen atoms (protons) and electrons "migrate" from one water molecule to the next, and the geometric structures in general, cause water to behave very differently than would be assumed according to the chemical and physical laws. However, to explain this would go beyond the scope of this book.

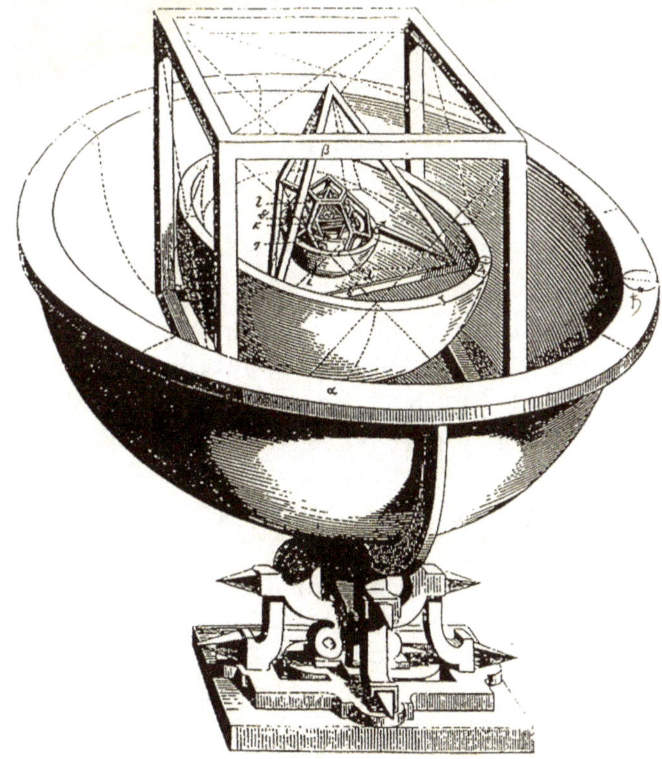

Fig. 7: The platonic solids: drawing by Johannes Kepler (1571 – 1630)

Weak compounds dissolve solid crystals

Water molecules are especially suitable for dissolving ionic compounds. Due to their different electrical charge, they can be inserted between the positively and negatively charged ions of an ion matrix, for example in a salt crystal, and surround the charged particles with a hydrate shell:

Common salt - sodium chloride NaCl - is a very strong compound when dry. If you put it in water, it is dissolved by the positively charged Na^+ connecting with the negative poles of the H_2O molecules and the negatively charged Cl^- connecting with the positive poles of the H_2O molecules.

As can be seen from this simple example, the weak compounds of the water molecules are able to dissolve strong and hard crystal compounds. So, water is a universal, natural solvent that can break strong and complex compounds. **These is one of the fundamental principles of chemical reactions**.

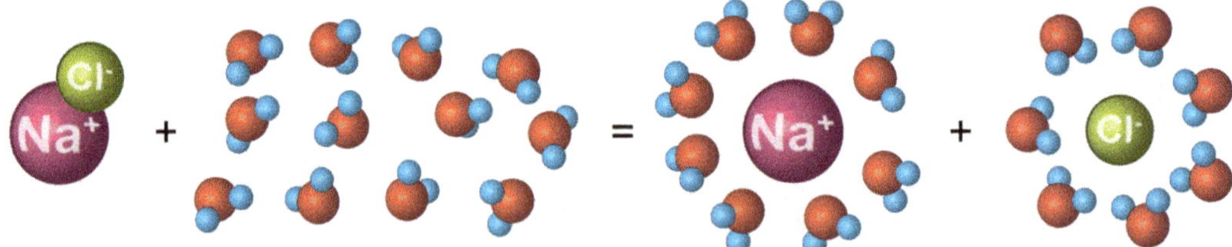

Fig. 8: Common salt NaCl and water are converted into dissolved Na⁺ and dissolved Cl⁻

Water as a solvent

Water therefore strives to dissolve the substances with which it comes in contact. The dissolving ability of water depends mainly on four factors:

- **The Temperature**: The higher the temperature of the water, the faster the water molecules move and the better substances are dissolved. For example, flavours and colorants of tea leaves dissolve better in hot than in cold water.

- **The difference in pH**: The greater the difference between the water's pH and the pH of the solute, the better it dissolves in water. For example, sodium bicarbonate dissolves better in acidic liquid, while a typical kidney stone is an oxalic acid crystal and dissolves in an alkaline liquid.

- **The saturation of water with dissolved substances**: The more substances are already dissolved in water; the less new substances can be dissolved. However, this effect is only relevant when the amount of dissolved substances approaches the saturation limit. Thus, salt dissolves well up to the saturation limit, only when the saturation limit is reached, no further salts can be dissolved. If the water then evaporates, salt crystals crystallize out.

- **The size of water clusters**: The smaller the water clusters are, the better they can dissolve substances, since water only reacts only at the surface of its water clusters. Smaller water clusters therefore have a larger surface area in relation to their volume. The cluster size can be influenced by various physical measures. Turbulence (mechanical or magnetic), free flow, evaporation, electrolysis and so on are ways to break up and minimize the cluster structures, while pressure – e.g. in pumps – and non-turbulent straight flow – e.g. in water pipes – weld clusters together and enlarge and immobilize them.

  For example, glacier water, water from a babbling brook, swirled water or ionised water from a water ioniser consist of small water clusters - this water is also called "hexagonal water". In contrast, water from a water pipe, for example from your kitchen faucet, has large water clusters and less solvent power.

These four parameters have different strong effects: temperature and pH-value difference are very important for the solubility, whereas saturation with dissolved substances is hardly relevant, because saturated solutions are rarely used as solvents, the cluster size is especially relevant for cold extracts and inside of organisms.

Water as information carrier

Water has different levels and scales in which it can react to external influences:

Undisputed, since determined by simple measuring instruments, are the state forms of water and the physical and chemical reactions and parameters, such as **temperature, surface tension, boiling point, freezing point, pH value, electrical charge** (redox value) and **conductivity** (dissolved minerals). Here, water reacts to the physical and chemical influences from the environment.

More difficult to determine, but still objectively measurable is the **cluster size** of water, which can be proven with modern NMR (Nuclear Magnetic Resonance) analysis.

Controversial and only explainable on the level of quantum physics, are the "esoteric" or "subtle" parameters, such as **direction of rotation, information content, vibrations** and so on. However, water molecules have at least four levels, in which information can be recorded, stored and transmitted:

The **first level of information** is **the frequency and the rhythm of the disintegration and new formation** of the hydrogen bonds between the individual water molecules in a water cluster, comparable to a three-dimensional, structured dance, in which the individual water molecules connect with ever new partners to "dance" a particular piece. It can be assumed that this "dance pattern" creates a three-dimensional frequency, that its rhythm can be shaped from the outside and that it can influence and structure the surrounding life in a living environment.

The **second level of information** lies in the **symmetry**: water is an asymmetrical, chiral molecule, which has a direction of rotation, a front and a back, right and left - just as there are, for example, right- and left-turning quartz crystals.

Quartz (silicon SiO_2) has a similar structure to water, but it is solid and its molecules are larger. Like water, quartz is transparent, refractive of light and reacts to electrical current.

Quartz crystals have various symmetries that can be measured and described:

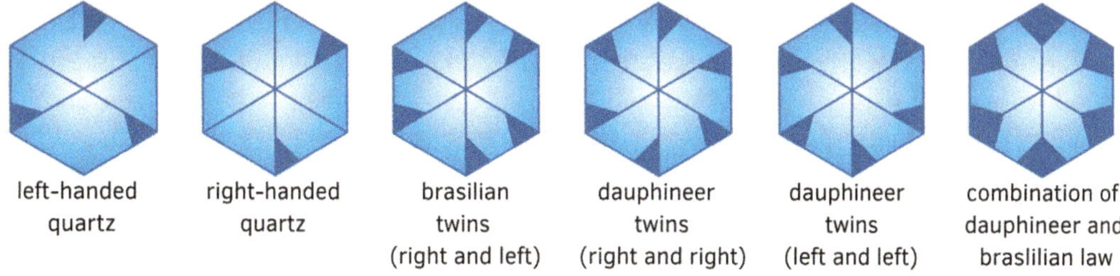

Fig. 9: Symmetries of quartz crystals

For quartz crystals this piezoelectric property is utilized technically, no computer would work without the use of SiO_2 oscillations: The crystal responds to pressure with an electric signal and to an electric signal with expansion or contraction.

The orientation of molecules in water clusters is a factor that can be assumed to have a major impact on biological microstructures – just as in technology, for example, it is only possible to work with pure either left- or right-rotating crystals, but these are rare, so that quartz crystals are synthetically produced for technical applications.

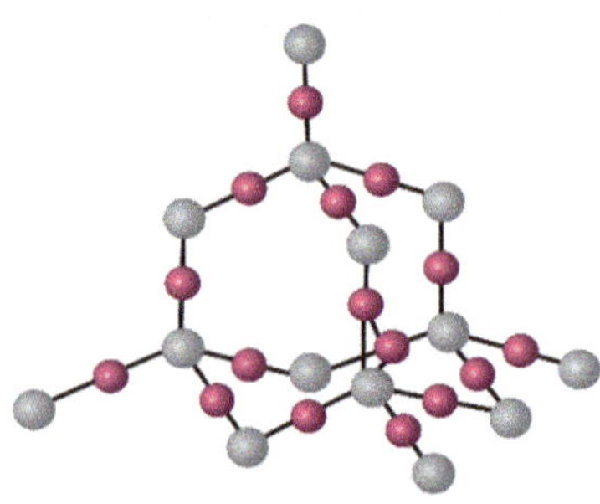

Fig. 10: The lattice structure of a quartz crystal (SiO₂)

Since the structure of silicon and minerals and crystals consisting mainly of silicon is so similar to the structure of water, resonances can occur between the oscillations of the silicon or quartz crystals and the oscillations of the water. Perhaps this is one of the reasons why silicon, the second most abundant element on earth, plays such a crucial role in our body for the structure of tissue and overall health.

The comparison with the SiO_2 molecule, the technical foundation of modern information technology, shows clearly which other information structures are still existing in the H_2O molecule, but cannot yet be measured objectively due to the inadequacy of the measurement technology.

The **third level of information** lies in the **oscillating structures** of the H_2O molecule. Since the H atoms do not form an exact tetrahedron angle with the O atom, they are always under tension and "oscillate". It is quite reasonable to assume that these oscillation structures are subject to certain order patterns, i.e. that they have an information content, and that these patterns can be influenced from the outside. So, it is physically conceivable that oscillation patterns from a chemical substance can be transmitted to the oscillations of the water molecules by intense turbulence (homeopathy) or by UV light or the electromagnetic force of the sun (Bach flower essence) and are permanently stored by the water molecules, or that the natural oscillation or the electric field of a living being or of a substance can influence the oscillation patterns of the water molecules.

The **fourth level of information** can be found in the **quantum physical structure of the atoms**, i.e. in the internal structure of the energy vortexes that form the quarks and thus the protons and neutrons of the atomic nuclei, as well as in the structure of the energy field between the atomic nuclei of the oxygen and the two hydrogen atoms and the electrons surrounding them. The way in which these energy vortexes and fields are formed, structured, informed and influenced has not yet been researched due to the lack of suitable measuring instruments. However, unbiased observations of the effects show that the theoretical considerations of quantum physics can explain phenomena in nature that cannot be explained otherwise.

For example, *Dr Huping Hu*, an American scientist, conducted the following experiment: He placed an airtight glass container with chloroform, a strong anaesthetic, between another airtight glass container filled with water, and a magnetic coil, with which he generated a pulsating magnetic field. When test persons drank from this water in a double-blind setting, it showed measurable effects such as those that occur when taking or inhaling anaesthetics. These effects were stronger with normal tap water than with distilled water, indicating that minerals in the water are necessary for information dissemination. The same effect also occurred when the closed glass with the anaesthetic was placed between the magnetic coil and the head of a test person.

These four information levels mentioned and explained here are not yet recognized in conventional science, but they all can all be explained with conventional or quantum physics.

I am convinced that sooner or later there will be methods to proof the existence and properties of these information levels with imaging techniques or perhaps even to measure physical values, and thus to explain the mode of action of homeopathy, Bach flower remedies, Reiki or healings by pure power of thought in a scientific-physical way.

World history in a water drop

Look at a drop of water. This water drop contains approx. 1.8×10^{15} (1,800,000,000,000,000) water molecules. Each of these water molecules has its own history, dating back to the time of the origin of the earth, carrying information, rhythms, frequencies and vibrations of millions of years, from glaciers and seas, from humans, animals and plants, from streams and rivers, from the soil and from the atmosphere around the globe. These water molecules come together and meet in a unique combination of oscillations, vibrations and "stories" in this single drop of water, which is unique and only exists once on Earth and will never exist again.

Maybe this "stories" are another reason that life is not possible without water?

Water molecules only become "new" and virtually "virgin" again when they are separated into their components hydrogen and oxygen and then "reassembled" again, as it happens for example in electrolysis, where hydrogen gas and oxygen gas are produced.

Water cycle and civilisation

Water evaporates and rises in the uppermost atmospheric layers, into stratosphere and troposphere. Where the force of gravity and air pressure are very low, the tiny water droplets are torn apart and separated into single water molecules. These individual water molecules are especially capable of absorbing the unfiltered radiation and frequencies of the sun and the cosmos. They absorb this solar and cosmic radiation and thereby shield the earth from them – water vapour is a far more effective "climate gas" than the much-criticised CO_2. Loaded with cosmic frequencies, they start the "return journey" to earth, gather in clouds and fall down in rain.

In recent decades, other, man-made frequencies have been added to the natural cosmic frequencies. From long-wave transmitters that can broadcast their frequencies from one location around the globe, and transmitters for influencing the weather such as the HAARP facilities in Alaska, Australia and elsewhere, trough satellite communications, radar, radio and television stations to short wave mobile communication transmitters, they all influence water molecules with a "salad" of different, mostly digitally modulated, unnatural frequencies.

Back on earth, water is supposed to seep into the soil or sink to the bottom of the oceans to be charged with the earth frequencies, in particular the Schumann frequency of 7.83 Hz. But even there is not spared from man-made interfering frequencies and electrical charges. On the shore, these interfering frequencies originate mainly from the global high-voltage grid, which is grounded in the groundwater and thus transmits the interference currents and frequencies into the water, but also from power lines and data cables buried in the ground. Power lines and data cables also pass through the oceans, and submarine communication frequencies affect the water, while the whale songs that traverse the water over hundreds of kilometres are becoming increasingly rare.

The impact of these man-made interfering frequencies on the water, on its properties and possibly on the entire life on earth has not yet been researched. Nor is it known how far life on earth depends on the cosmic, solar and earth frequencies transported by the water.

Make water information visible

Various so-called "imaging methods" such as the Drop Picture Method, Capillary Dynamolysis, Biocrystallisation or Ice Crystal Method make it possible to visualize "information" and structures of water as a qualitative, pictorial statement.

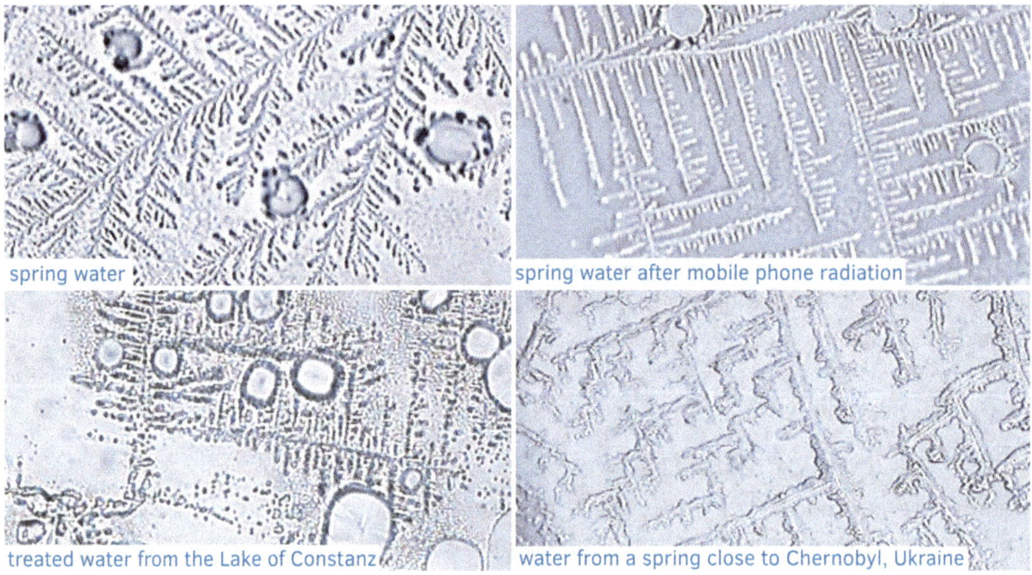

Fig. 11: Biocrystallisation images to assess the quality of the water structure
Images by Praxislabor Dr Hoefer, Ueberlingen, Germany (www.praxislabor-hoefer.de)

Healing with water information

Ancient healers already used water information for healing purposes: Hildegard von Bingen (1098-1179) recommended to place certain stones and crystals in water and then drink it. Paracelsus (1494-1541) distinguished between different oscillating waters with different characteristics and properties. Jakob Lorber (1800-1864) advised exposing sick people to the sun and giving them spring water irradiated by the sun to drink. The homeopathy developed by Samuel Hahnemann (1755-1843) is a result of this centuries-old knowledge.

Chapter 2: Biological correlations

The human body consists of about 60 to 70% of water, more in youth and less in old age. Water is essential for the functioning of life processes. Whoever takes a holistic view of mankind must necessarily pay the utmost attention to water. Approximately one-fifth of the water in the human body – at a body weight of 80 kg this is about 50 litres – is found as an intercellular fluid (between the cells), the so-called lymph. More than half is bound as cell water in the cells, the remainder is found in the blood and in the organs. Without water, no life processes can take place.

Man is an aquarium

The lymph is virtually a copy of the primordial ocean in which life originated many millions of years ago. This primordial ocean was a salty sea with **0.9% salinity** - slightly lower than today. At that time, individual cells formed cell clusters that started to organize themselves and to develop a kind of intelligence, from which the mammals finally emerged. We find this primordial ocean environment again in our lymph – the value of 0.9% salinity is well known as physiological saline solution. The lymph surrounds all cells and contains, besides water and salts, trace elements and protein. It is the "milieu" in which cells are "dwelling" and part of the connective tissue. If the cell milieu is not optimal, the cells cannot develop in a healthy way.

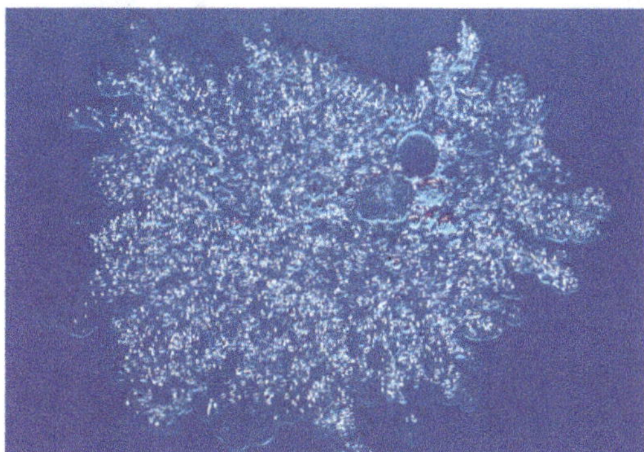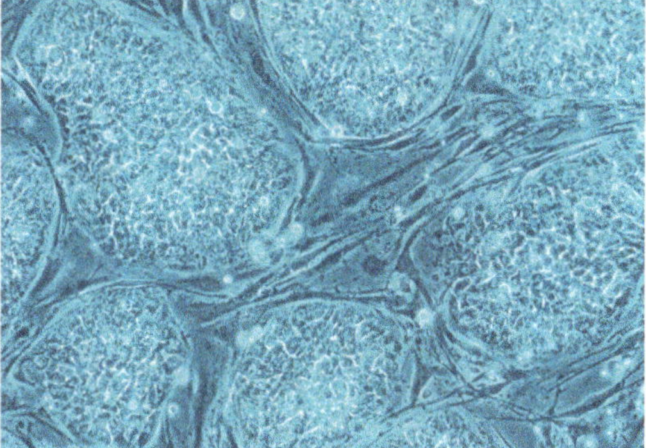

Fig. 12: There are clear similarities between amoebae (left) and mammalian (right) cells. Images by Arthur Hauck (left), Nissim Benvenisty (right)

Therefore, we can compare our body with an aquarium: Our body cells are aquatic creatures that live in the lymphatic sea, from which they feed themselves and which absorbs the waste products of their metabolism. In an aquarium, the health of the "inhabitants" depends above all on the quality of the food and the cleanliness of the water. No aquarium owner would give medicines to sick fish, instead he would control the quality of the water, change the water and ensure a healthy feeding.

The lymph

While blood and blood circulation are well known and well-studied, the lymphatic system is still a closed book even for many doctors. The "conventional" medicine only focuses on the "substances" in the human being, disorders of the whole organism are attributed to deficiency symptoms or incorrect distribution of these "substances". The water in the body – whether in the connective tissue as lymph, in the blood or in the cells – is only considered to be a "filler", a neutral transport medium at best, but not a carrier of information and properties, whose quality is essential for the health of the entire organism.

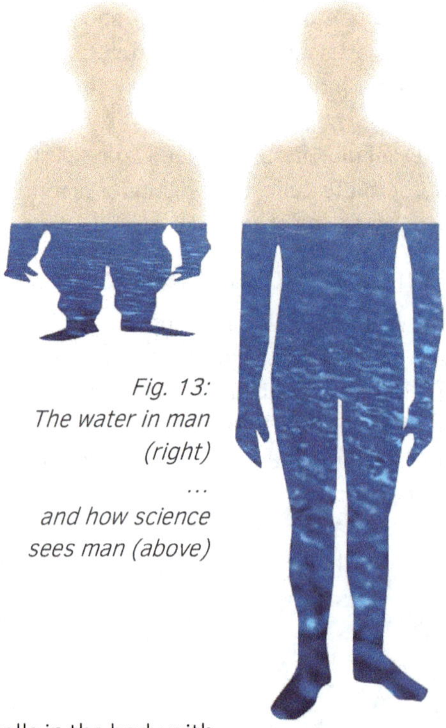

However, the quality, properties and composition of the lymph are essential for overall function, immune status, nutrient supply and waste transport in our body. It determines cell health and the longevity of the body's cells, as an experiment conducted by the Medicine Nobel Prize laureate *Alexis Carrell* (1873-1944) shows: He kept a chicken heart cell alive for 28 years by exchanging the surrounding fluid daily.

Fig. 13:
The water in man
(right)
…
and how science
sees man (above)

Water molecules of the lymph surround proteins and cells in the body with a hydrate layer. Korean research shows a structure of water surrounding living proteins and cells in the body in three layers:

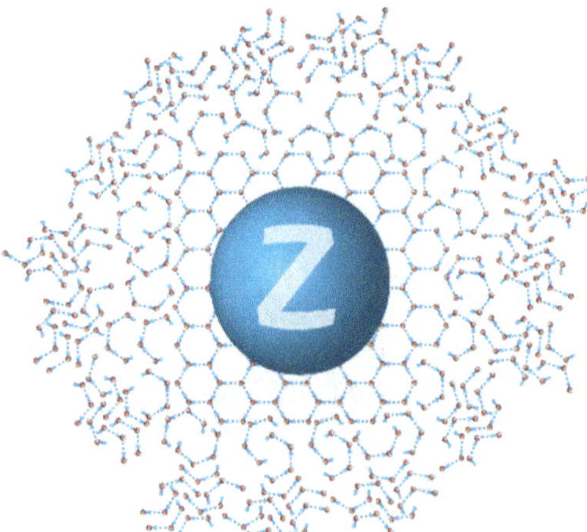

Fig. 14: Water structures around a body cell (Z)

The innermost layer – some water molecules strong – is structured like a liquid ice crystal, with larger hollow spaces like "liquid" water.

The second layer still has slightly crystal-like structures.

The third layer corresponds to "normal" lymph water, its resonance frequency of 53 Hz is measured in the nuclear resonance method when a living body cell is measured.

This "outermost" water layer is followed by the "normal" salty lymphatic fluid.

The water"cycle" in the body of man

Water passes through mouth, the oesophagus and the stomach into the small intestine – preferably in the morning, the best drinking time, because then the stomach is empty and a relatively thin tube (if you have not eaten a heavy and oily steak the evening before), the gastric acid-producing parietal cells on the gastric wall have not yet received any taste signal from the taste buds in the mouth and are still "sleeping", and so the water is allowed to pass through by the pylorus, the gatekeeper, which "guards" the exit of the stomach towards the intestine – provided that it is pure water without additives, because only water without additives does not irritate the taste buds in the mouth and does not have to be "pre-treated" in the stomach. This is how water gets into the small intestine. If the stomach is full, only a small portion of the water can pass above the acidic food chyme and reaches the pylorus unadulterated, the rest mixes with the gastric acid.

The small intestinal flora needs to be sufficiently hydrated by neutral or slightly alkaline water, because the "good" bacteria in the small intestine need sufficient moisture and a slightly alkaline environment. Especially if the pancreas, with its strong alkaline secretion intended to neutralize the acidic food chyme and raise its pH to the alkaline range, is overstrained or damaged (as it is usually the case with diabetics, for example), the small intestine environment needs support from neutral or alkaline water.

Water is absorbed in the small intestine via the intestinal villi. In these villi, a blood vessel and a lymph vessel are located in parallel under the permeable mucous membrane. Interestingly, the intestinal mucosa has a **positive electrical charge**, therefore attracting negatively charged molecules and repelling positively charged molecules. This is necessary because all molecules originating from plant and vegetable food, the primordial food of man, are negatively charged or have negatively charged ends and can thus be attracted by the positively charged intestinal mucosa. The positive charge of the intestinal mucosa also

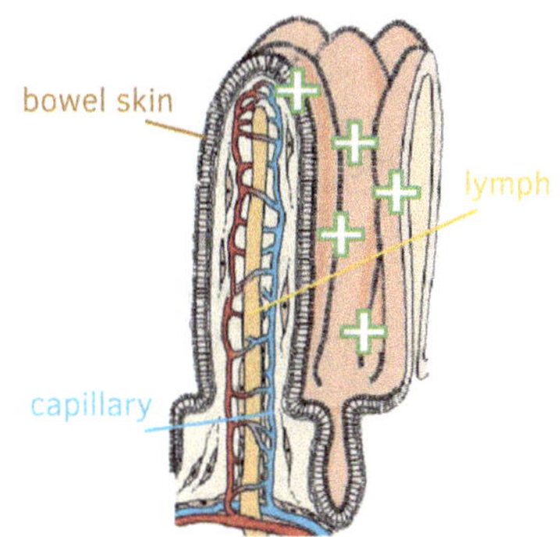

Fig. 15: Intestinal villi

explains why non-ionised alkaline, positively charged minerals dissolved in water, such as we find as Calcium Ca^{++} or Magnesium Mg^+ in mineral water, cannot be absorbed, whereas they can be absorbed when embedded in organic molecules.

Through the permeable intestinal mucosa, sugar and amino acids are absorbed and carried away by the blood vessels, water and fats are absorbed and transported by the lymph vessels. Sugar and amino acids pass through the portal vein to the liver, where toxins are filtered out, water and fat pass through the lymph nodes, also filtering out toxins and acids, into the mammary duct, which is fed into the left jugular vein and thus into the bloodstream, In this way, the water becomes blood serum and "dilutes" the blood, afterwards, through the exchange in the capillaries, it returns to the body as lymph.

By understanding these processes, it is becoming clear that

- the lymph nodes in the abdomen are crucial for the immune system,
- the immune system is alleviated when water is consumed as neutral or slightly alkaline water,
- the pH of drinking water affects the pH of the lymph and blood serum,
- inorganic minerals dissolved in water are difficult or impossible to absorb.

In our body's water balance, the "endogenous" or oxidation water, being produced during the production of energy in the mitochondria by the fusion of hydrogen and oxygen, must not be forgotten - for an adult person it is about 300 ml daily.

Transport"systems" in the body

Basically, there are two types of transport systems in the human body:

Active transport takes place via the **blood. Regulated and pulsated** by the heart (the fact that the heart is not a pump is not only confirmed by calculations of its performance, but also by recent scientific research, which shows through flow patterns on living hearts that the blood in the heart flows in vortexes in all phases and is by no means "squeezed" through the arteries by the power of the heart muscles), the blood actively distributes sugar, oxygen, hormones, messenger substances etc. throughout the body. Blood consists mainly of blood serum that is formed from the lymph and returns to it.

Next to the red blood cells carrying oxygen, the blood also contains white blood cells, the "body police", which form oxygen radicals if necessary – e.g. during infections –, oxidizing foreign and harmful bacteria or viruses (e.g. rob them of their electrons and burning them). Through the blood, the "body intelligence" can distribute messenger substances from endocrine glands throughout the body in no time at all – e.g. stress hormones, happiness hormones and so on.

Through the blood, all these substances are brought into the capillaries. These thinnest and finest veins are permeable – like the intestinal mucosa –, allowing oxygen, nutrients, hormones, etc. to pass into the intercellular space and the lymph and reach the body cells. The gaseous waste, especially CO_2, is also absorbed by the blood and transported to the lungs. If you enter a bedroom in the morning after somebody slept in it with locked windows, you can smell the sour gases excreted during the night.

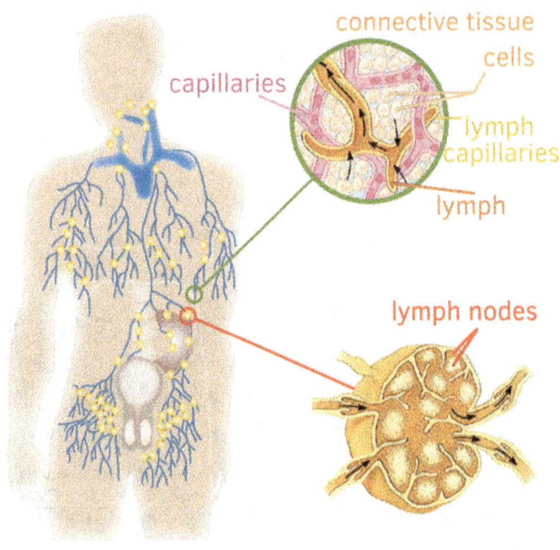

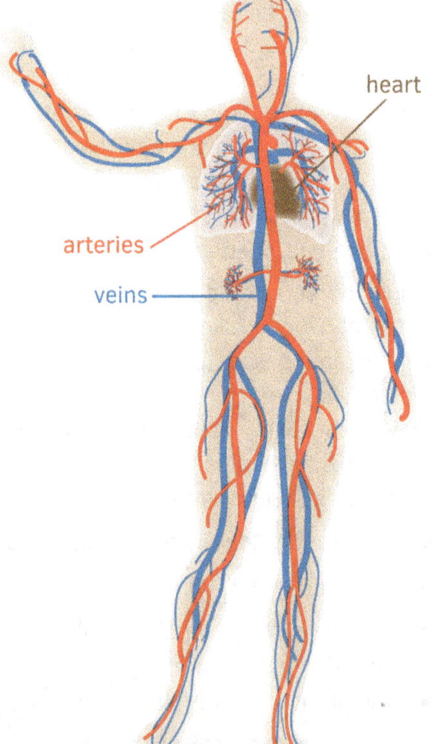

Fig. 16 (top): The lymphatic system

Fig. 17 (right): The blood system

The **lymph** flows through the intercellular space, where it takes over the second part of the transport chain, the "last mile" to its destination, the body cells, as well as the disposal of the waste produced in the cells and in the tissues. This is a **passive transport**, i.e. there is no channelled flow of substances, no carrier, but the distribution of substances takes place according to the **laws of diffusion and concentration equalisation**, which means they move from places of high concentration to places of low concentration until the concentration is equalized.

Apart from water, the lymph consists of dissolved salts and protein in varying proportions depending on the body region. The more acidic the lymphatic water is, the more gel-like the contained protein becomes. Gel-like protein in turn affects the fluidity and permeability of the lymph for diffusion processes.

Speaking about "**hyperacidity**", which is often held responsible for more or less all diseases, it becomes obvious here that this "hyperacidity" refers exclusively to the pH in the connective tissue and in the lymph system, because "acidic" is not "bad" per se, but essential and vital in some organs and parts of our body.

80% of the lymphatic fluid is located in the abdominal cavity, the stomach area, since here, with the food, most foreign substances and thus most dangers for the body health arrive. In the abdominal cavity, the centre of our immune system and health is located – a healthy intestine, which can digest food without producing fusel alcohols, fermentation and decay processes, is therefore of utmost importance not only for overall health in general, but also for the function of the immune system, as a prevention against allergies etc.

Our body cells do not have a direct connection to blood capillaries, just as your property has no direct highway access. This results in an increased concentration of oxygen, nutrients and sugar in the connective tissue and lymph around the capillaries, while around the cells there is an increased concentration of carbonic acid – carbon dioxide CO_2 dissolved in water – and other waste products of cell metabolism. As the cells consume oxygen and sugar, a suction effect and a concentration gradient develops, oxygen and nutrients migrate towards the cells, while carbon dioxide and the other gaseous acids migrate towards the capillaries to be absorbed by the blood and transported away to be exhaled through the lungs. *(See also Fig. 27, page 35)*

The other waste and residual substances of the cell metabolism are gradually channelled into the lymphatic system and its vessels, where they dissolve in the lymph fluid, which is moved by light pumping movements of surrounding muscles, cleaned by lymph nodes and finally fed back into the bloodstream via the superior vena cava. Thus, the **lymphatic circulation blood serum – lymph – blood serum** is completed. The functionality of these transport chains is crucial for the health, longevity and performance of the cells.

Medical Nobel Prize laureate *Alexis Carrel*, who kept a chicken heart alive for 28 years by regularly changing the surrounding nutrient solution, said: *"The cell is immortal. It is simply the fluid in which it floats that degrades. By replacing this fluid at regular intervals, we will give the cell what it needs to nourish itself and, as far as we know, the pulse of life can continue indefinitely"*.

By understanding these processes, it is becoming clear that

- the passive transport in the lymph has an important function in the body,
- a low pH lymphatic fluid is more viscous and gel-like due to coagulated proteins than a high pH lymphatic fluid,
- the consistency and fluidity of the lymph have a direct effect on the supply and disposal of the cells.

Alkaline and acidic: the digestive system

The food we eat is processed by bacteria in the digestive system in such a way that the substances needed by our body can be absorbed by the mucous membranes, mainly in the small intestine. Hence many trillions of bacteria live more or less symbiotically together with us.

Each type of bacteria has an optimal environment in terms of temperature, pH, humidity ..., in which it can thrive and work best. Our digestive system is designed to always provide the bacteria that are important for the respective digestive process with the optimal habitat. The digestive system is therefore divided into four sections with different pH values:

- The **oral cavity** is the part of our body most densely populated by bacteria. It should be slightly alkaline to allow the good bacterial flora to develop and to keep the bad bacteria such as caries in check. Thus, saliva should always be slightly alkaline, which is achieved by an alkaline lymphatic fluid with alkaline enzymes, from which saliva is produced.

- The **stomach** is very acidic. Its low pH and its high chlorine content help to break down proteins and to "disinfect" the food by killing food-borne bacteria, fungi and other microorganisms. To reach this acidic pH value, the parietal cells on the stomach wall take the chlorine (Cl) from the NaCl (common salt) dissolved in the blood to form hydrochloric acid HCl, which has a pH of around pH 2.

- The **small intestine** should be alkaline again in order to be able to provide optimal habitat for the alkaline-loving bacteria that are able to break down and digest our food. In the small intestine, the bacteria do the main digestive work. To neutralize the sour chyme, the excretory ducts of the liver, bile and pancreas lead to the beginning of the small intestine and bring alkaline secretions with them, which the pancreas produces with sodium hydroxide (NaOH) from the sodium in the blood.

- The **large intestine** is again slightly acidic, as minerals are absorbed through its mucous membrane and dead bacteria are neutralized and digested by other bacteria.

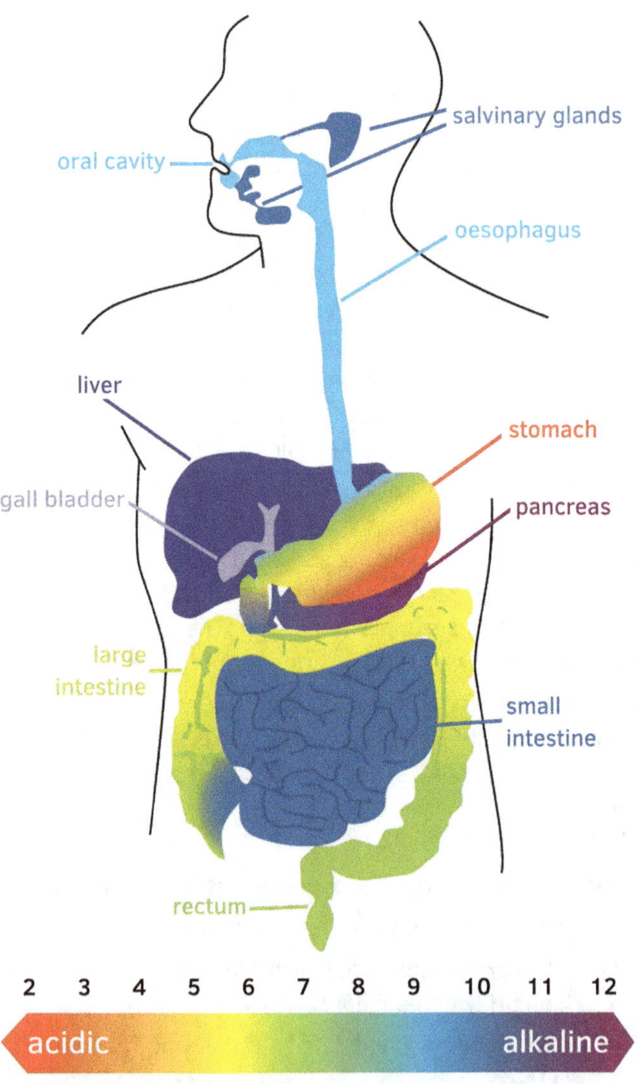

Fig. 18: pH values in the body

Supply and waste disposal in the body cell

Like unicellular organisms living in water, the health of our cells depends primarily on the fluid surrounding them. Apart from specialized tasks, energy production is their main duty. What we call "life", it happens in the cell.

The energy production takes place in the 1,000 to 6,000 **mitochondria** located in every body cell, which are the power stations of our body. Inside the mitochondria, hydrogen is extracted from carbohydrates and fatty acids in the so-called "citric acid cycle". The hydrogen is stored in the coenzyme NADH and then oxidized with oxygen, which diffuses from the lymph

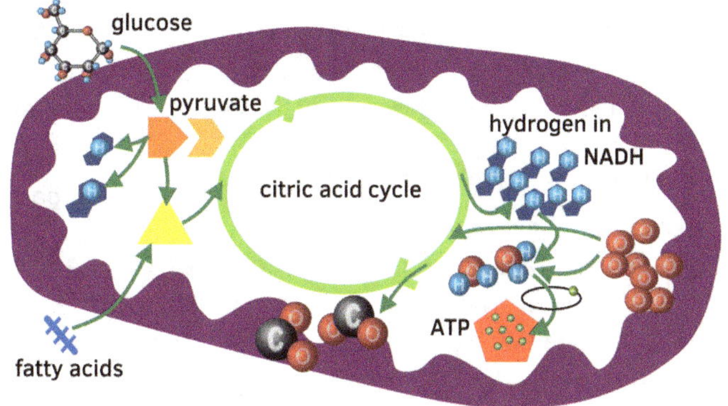

Fig. 19: Energy production inside of a mitochondrion

into the cell through channels in the cell wall. This oxidation produces energy – like in a fuel cell – that charges the enzyme AMP (adenosine monophosphate) to ATP (adenosine tri-phosphate), which distributes energy throughout the cell and returns as AMP. This oxidation also produces the so-called endogenous or oxidation water, which contributes to the water supply to the cell.

The carbon from the carbohydrates which is no longer needed – it becomes carbonic acid in combination with water – and all other impurities that enter the cells with the carbohydrates and fatty acids are what is called "slags", unspecified toxins, in alternative medicine. They lower the pH inside the cell, so in a working cell the cell water is always slightly acidic. However, these acids must be continuously removed so that the acid concentration in the cell does not raise too high. For de-acidification, the acids are transported through channels through the cell wall into the connective tissue fluid. To prevent the cell from drying out, the cell water must be replaced, therefore, slightly alkaline, clean water should re-enter the cell as easily as possible.

This water supply to the cells is provided by special water channels that are lined with **aquaporins**, positively charged, spiral-shaped proteins. They allow only negatively charged water molecules to enter the cell, preventing positively charged, low-energy water neutralizing the electrical energy generated in the cell. In 2003, the American physician *Peter Agre* was awarded the Nobel Prize in Chemistry in 2003 for his research on the functions of aquaporins.

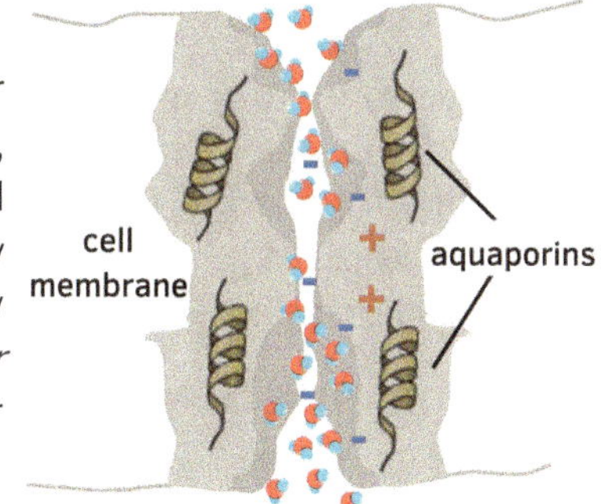

Fig. 20: aquaporins

Thus, a cell may dry out, even though there is enough water stored in the connective tissues, if this connective tissue water is positively charged. In a dried-up cell, toxins can no longer be removed properly, the cell becomes acidified, and energy production is impaired because there is not enough oxygen available for combustion, as it is "swallowed" by excess acid. If a cell is persistently over-acidified and therefore there is permanently too little oxygen available, the sugar begins to ferment and the cell converts its metabolism from the aerobic (oxygen-requiring) to the anaerobic energy production. In this state, the natural control mechanisms of a cell are overridden and it begins to grow uncontrollably – the first stage of cancer development.

By understanding these processes, it is becoming clear that

- a cell always produces acidic slags or „toxins"
- only an alkaline cell environment can properly absorb these acidic slags from the cell
- a cell dries up if there is no "good" negatively charged water around
- cell fermentation – identified as the cause of cancer by the Nobel laureate Otto Warburg in 1967 – is caused by an acid rather than an alkaline lymphatic fluid.

Water deployment in the body

Water is not evenly distributed in the body. The water content ranges from 96% in the eyes to 10% in the teeth. The lymphatic fluid consists of about 90%, the blood about 88% of water.

Looking at the adjacent table, it becomes obvious that "living" and "conscious" organs contain a high percentage of water, while in "dead" and unconsciously working organs, the water content is low.

The water distribution in our body shows that water is the carrier of life and consciousness - or at least necessary for a conscious being!

Organ	Water content in %
Eye	94 - 96%
Brain	91 - 93%
Heart	approx. 79%
Lungs	approx. 78%
Muscles	approx. 76%
Liver	approx. 72%
Skin	approx. 70%
Cartilage	50 - 60%
Hair and Nails	20 - 30%
Bones	20 - 22%
Adipose tissue	10 - 20%
Teeth	approx. 10%

Tab 1: Water content of various organs

Excursus: history of evolution

From generation to generation, genetic predispositions of humans change only in a very small per thousand range, our genetic predispositions originate largely from the Stone Age. For hundreds of thousands of years, Homo sapiens lived in caves or in the jungle.

The daily routine of a Stone Age hunter or gatherer was quite simple: In the morning, drinking water was the first thing to do, therefore, the caves or sleeping quarters had to be located on streams or water courses to have water sufficiently available. Afterwards, the food for the day had to be collected or hunted with high physical effort, until – at noon at the earliest, usually only in the evening – it was time for eating and then – in absence of television or cultural program – for sleeping. Our internal clock is set to this rhythm: Our ingestion and digestive system "sleeps" from about 4 to 12 a.m., the ingestion phase is from 12 a.m. to 8 p.m., the processing phase from 8 p.m. to 4 a.m.

Recommendation: The order of food intake

Fermentation processes in stomach and intestine are the causes of many complaints. They are mainly caused by wrong food combinations and sequences. It is important to eat "faster" food – i.e. food passing the stomach and the intestines in a shorter time – before food that need to stay longer in the stomach and the intestines for digestion.

The order of food intake should be: carbohydrates before proteins before fat – and well chewed before quickly engulfed. For example, if you eat a fruit salad after a fatty roast with an oily sauce, the fruits are "trapped" for up to nine hours at optimal fermentation temperatures behind the meat – with corresponding consequences: Acids and alcohols are formed which acidify the small intestine and can lead to a measurable blood alcohol level.

Chapter 3: Oxidation and Reduction Reactions

Oxidation and reduction are the most important reactions in biological systems. Oxidation and reduction of molecules and the resulting flow of electrons = energy are the foundation of every human life, but also of life in general. In chemistry, oxidation is defined as the release of electrons (e.g. rusting metal), reduction is defined as the absorption of electrons.

Oxidation = Donation of electrons   **Reduction = Uptake of electrons**

Oxidation and reduction always take place simultaneously. The ability of a substance to release or accept electrons is called **redox potential**. The release of an electron (oxidation) sets energy free from the oxidized molecule – its redox potential becomes more positive –, the acceptance of an electron (reduction) stores energy in the reduced molecule – its redox potential becomes more negative.

The redox potential of a substance is measured in mV (millivolt) – a negative value means an excess of negative charge = electrons = energy, a positive value an excess of positive charge = lack of electrons = lack of energy. The terminology used here is irritating, since a positive (good) fact, namely a surplus of energy, an excess of electrons, is called "negative". It dates back to the early days of static electricity research, when the discovery of frictional electricity was based on the assumption that the charge of glass was positive and that electricity would transfer from glass to other materials. Only later was it understood that the electrons flow from the (so defined) negative pole to the positive pole. Therefore, electrons are given a negative sign.

A e$^-$		**B**		**A**		**B e$^-$**
Electron donor	+	Electron acceptor	=	oxidizes (is losing an e$^-$)	+	reduces (is gaining an e$^-$)

When an electron-rich molecule A comes into contact with an electron-deficient molecule B, the following happens:

- **Molecule A** gives an electron e$^-$ to molecule B, the redox potential of A is increasing.
- **Molecule A is oxidized.**
- **Molecule B** receives an electron e$^-$ from molecule A, the redox potential of B is decreasing.
- **Molecule B is reduced.**

Redox reactions in our body – fundamentals of life

Man is a bioelectric being; electrons control and enable all our body actions, processes and reactions. Every process in the body – not only energy production – can be seen as an oxidation-reduction reaction, as electrons are passed from one molecule to another, first reducing and then re-oxidizing every molecule. Every movement, every thought, every process in our body – from breathing to trembling, from intestinal movement to muscle contraction, from heartbeat to speech – is caused by electrical signals emanating from the body's cells, whether controlled and consciously – like the sensory impressions of seeing, hearing, feeling, tasting – or unconsciously – like the heartbeat or the control of our digestive organs, salivary glands, stomach, pancreas, liver, etc. These signals ensure that every organ, every gland, every cell and every muscle involved does the right thing and produce the right "secretions" at the right time.

Energy transformation

Since we consume chemically bound energy like carbohydrates and sugars, fats or proteins, but need bioelectric energy to sustain life, we can call ourselves a "hybrid", burning chemical energy as "fuel" to produce bioelectric energy needed for our body to function.

Before we can consume them, carbohydrates, sugars, fats and proteins are produced in the **chlorophyll** of plants, utilizing water H_2O, carbon dioxide CO_2 and minerals from the soil. These reactions take place with the help of **photon energy** from sunlight, releasing oxygen O_2. The so produced carbohydrate, sugar, fat and protein molecules contain more energy = electrons than the CO_2 and H_2O from which they originate, they have been reduced because they have absorbed electrons.

In humans and mammals, the conversion of chemical into bioelectric energy takes place in the **mitochondria** in the body cells. There, sugar and fat molecules are broken down in the citric acid cycle into their basic building blocks in order to release the hydrogen H contained in them. The hydrogen then reacts with oxygen O in a multi-stage process – similar to a fuel cell – to form water. During this process, energy = electrons are released. These electrons charge the enzyme adenosine mono-phosphate (AMP) to become an electrically negatively charged adenosine tri-phosphate (ATP), which contains excess electrons and acts as "messenger", bringing the energy to the places in the cell where it is needed. (*See also Fig. 19, page 21*)

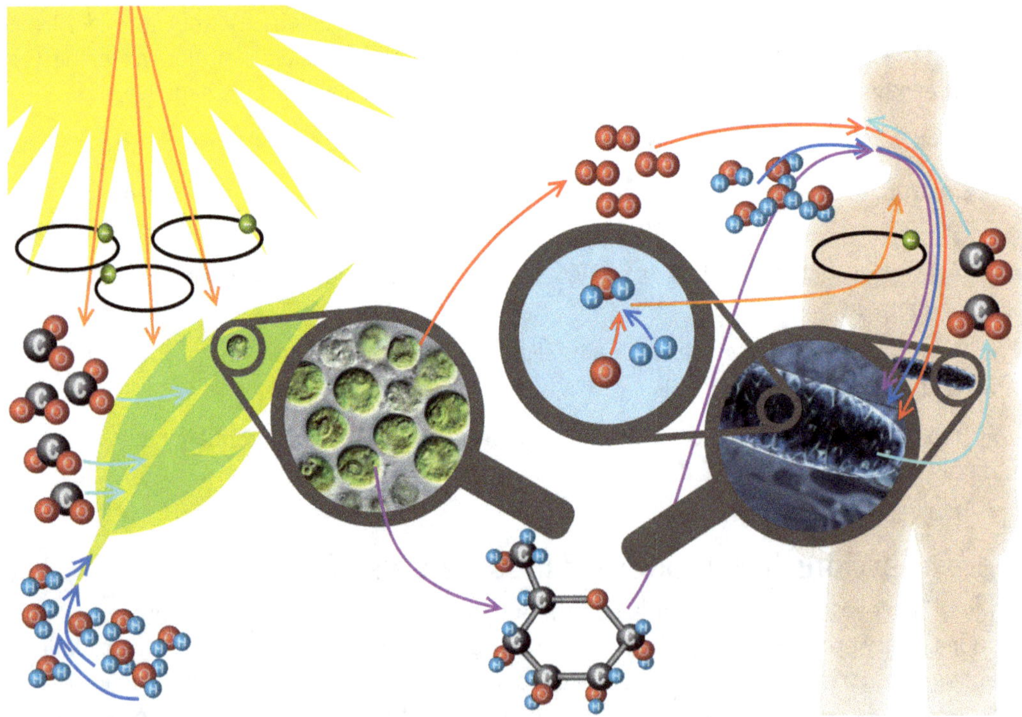

Fig. 21: The cycle of life: In the chlorophyll of plants, starch / sugar and oxygen are produced from water and carbon dioxide with the help of solar energy. In the mitochondria, hydrogen is extracted from the sugar, it reacts with oxygen to water, releasing the stored energy.

Vital oxygen

Oxygen is indispensable for the energy generating process, because the energy is generated through the oxidation of hydrogen extracted from food, forming water as the result. Water can therefore also be regarded as "oxidized di-hydrogen". The task of the oxygen is to release stored energy = electrons – no matter if this happens in a controlled and gentle process like in the mitochondria or in a violent and impetuous process like in a fire. Oxygen is the most important oxidizing agent for biological processes. Its concentration in the atmosphere of 21% is ideally and precisely balanced for life on earth.

A lower oxygen content in the air would inhibit oxidation processes and thus life; at a higher concentration, oxidation and combustion processes would take place spontaneously, and only charred matter would be left behind. As we can see, oxygen has an ambivalent role: On the one hand it is vital for life, because only with its help the hydrogen extracted from the storage molecules can be oxidized to release the energy it contains, on the other hand, like all other oxidizing agents, it damages other molecules. Without oxygen there is no life for higher organisms.

In the air, oxygen is relatively stable, because it exists as molecule O_2 and its two atoms form a common electron shell. In the body, oxygen is absorbed by the lungs, passes through the pulmonary alveoli into the blood and then through the connective tissue into the body cells, where it is needed for our energy production. Only in the **aerobic metabolism**, carbohydrates can be effectively broken down into carbon dioxide CO_2 and water to release energy. In case of oxygen deficiency, the body can resort to an **anaerobic** (without oxygen) conversion of the carbohydrates, which is inefficient and leaves behind more acidic waste products and toxins, which can lead to muscle soreness if, for example, the muscles are subjected to excessive strain.

Too much of a good thing?

The reaction between oxygen and the hydrogen bound in the NADH (see chapter *"Supply and waste disposal of the body cell"*) is vulnerable to malfunctions, not only because it takes place so often, but also because the quantity ratio between hydrogen and oxygen – two atoms of hydrogen to one atom of oxygen – must be exactly right at all times. If two hydrogen atoms are not available and ready for each oxygen atom, so-called **reactive oxygen species** ROS are formed – this happens to about 2% of the molecules at rest, during extreme physical effort by untrained people or during hyperventilation to up to 20%.

However, oxygen radicals can also develop as a result of UV or microwave radiation, burns or chemical reactions, for example at heavy metal molecules etc. In technology, oxygen radicals like hydrogen peroxide or ozone are helpful for disinfection.

Electrons always occur in pairs. Each electron has its "opponent". If this is missing, the unpaired electron reacts with neighbouring molecules to "procure" the missing electron.

ROS are the main cause of physical damage and involved in most diseases. ROS damage cells through oxidation, rob them of energy by stealing their electrons and make them susceptible to attack by bacteria or viruses. Oxygen radicals trigger chain reactions: It oxidizes molecule one, this oxidizes molecule two, this again molecule three ... and so on. This can also result in damage to the genetic material.

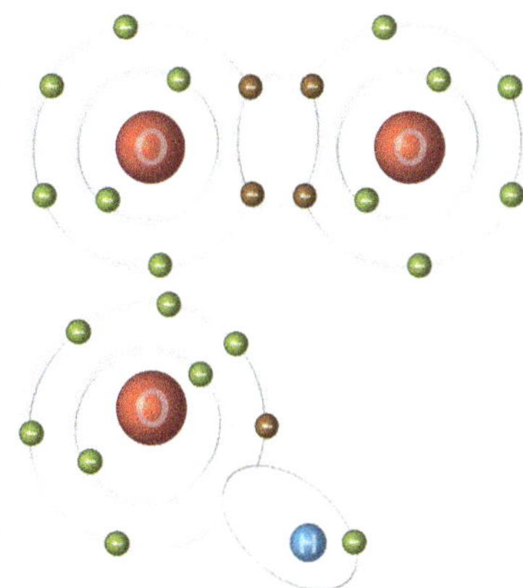

Fig. 22: An oxygen molecule (top) and an ROS (hydroxyl ion, bottom). Red: Unpaired electrons

Free radicals and antioxidants

We are exposed to a constant encounter with various microorganisms and live in continuous exchange with them. Especially in the mouth and in the intestines, there are large numbers of bacteria and other microorganisms, taking care for the digestion and decomposition of food.

In order to keep the growth of unwanted microorganisms in check, the defence system of our body forms neutrophils, a type of leukocyte, white blood cells. These neutrophils produce free radicals that can oxidize undesirable microorganisms. These so-called **primary free radicals** are the "weapons" of our immune system and are necessary for human survival. They must not be confused with **secondary free radicals**, the above-mentioned ROS, which are caused by excessive oxidation, incorrect breathing, etc. and damage our body.

In figurative terms, the primary radicals produced by the body's immune system and used to fight bacteria and viruses can be compared with the police or a regular army, while the secondary free radicals, the ROS, can be compared to terrorists eager to damage the body.

As the name suggests, antioxidants are substances that can act "against" oxidation. These are mainly vitamins, but also other substances of plant origin – like OPC – or animal origin such as Astaxanthin. Antioxidants have a "loose" electron with which they can reduce the oxidizing substance, i.e. they release their electron to the oxidizing substance. Unfortunately, antioxidants cannot distinguish between (harmful) secondary radicals (ROS) and the (useful) primary radicals of the immune system. Therefore, scientists warn against excessive intake of antioxidants, especially of synthetic origin. However, vitamins and other antioxidants have many other important tasks in the body in addition to their antioxidant effect – they are not considered essential for life for nothing. Therefore, it is not intended to warn against a diet rich in (natural) vitamins and antioxidants, but only against excessive consumption of isolated high-dose synthetic antioxidants.

Hydrogen

Hydrogen is the "partner" of oxygen in the water molecule. Like Yin and Yang, they embody the opposites, but together they constitute a whole. Their fusion is the cleanest form of energy generation – it takes place in our body and in technology as fuel cell technology.

Albert Szent-Gyorgyi, the Hungarian Nobel Prize winner in medicine (1937), recognised the importance of hydrogen for mankind.

As the smallest of all elements, it is so tiny that it can penetrate all cells, crossing also the blood-brain barrier. Although hydrogen is not an antioxidant, it has a similar effect to ROS. Hydrogen combines with such an ROS to form water H_2O, thus neutralizing it without leaving any residues at all.

Redox reactions in nature and technology

After **combustion**, the best known technical redox reaction is certainly **rusting**. While combustion is a sudden reaction of mostly organic substances with oxygen, rusting is a comparatively slow oxidation. Electrons are removed from the metal so that the cohesion of the iron atom is broken up and water can accumulate. Besides the protection against water and acids, a so-called sacrificial anode is a common and safe method to protect iron or steel against rust. This is used mainly on ships sailing in salt water: A piece of non-ferrous metal, usually zinc, is screwed to the ship's hull so that a voltage flows between the iron and the zinc, the zinc block slowly dissolves in the water and electrons flow from the zinc into the iron. As a result, the ship's iron hull always has a surplus of electrons and cannot rust.

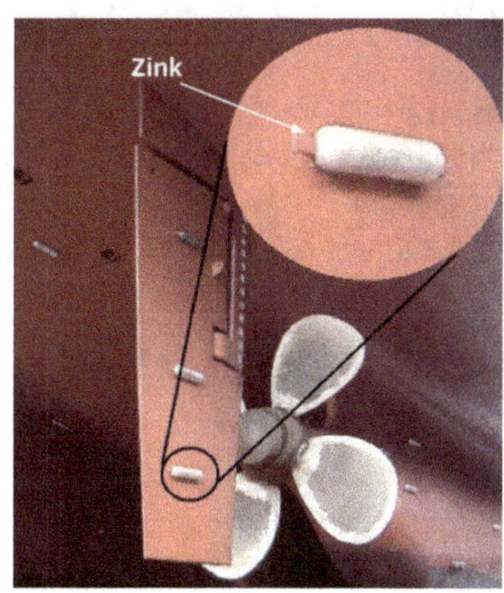

Fig. 23: New sacrificial anodes at a ship hull

A very strong redox reaction occurs, for example, with thermite, a mixture of powdered iron and aluminium. Due to the extremely high redox potential between these two metals, this powder can be ignited and burns at well over 2,000°C. It is used, for example, for welding railway sleepers because it liquefies steel very fast.

Redox values of our foods

Each substance has an electrical potential compared to another substance, i.e. a difference in electrical charge. This is called the oxidation-reduction-potential or ORP.

This ORP is usually measured in relation to the so-called standard hydrogen electrode, which is regarded as a "zero value". An ORP, as measured in mV (millivolt), is therefore never an absolute value, but describes the difference in electrical charge between two substances or – unless otherwise noted – between a substance and the standard hydrogen electrode.

The measurement of different foods gives the following result:

Foods	ORP values
Acetic acid 5%	+ 400 mV (±15)
Caffeinated lemonade	+ 300 mV (±25)
Tap water	+150 mV to +300 mV
Apple Juice	+112 mV (±15)
Beer	+74 mV (±15)
Coffee	+70 mV (±15)
Black Tea	+65 mV (±15)
Red Vine	+50 mV (±15)
Tomato juice	+36 mV (±15)
Green Tea (organic)	+30 mV (±15)
Dissolved Vitamin C	+30 mV to -30 mV
Dissolved Vitamin C plus Iron	+30 mV to -70 mV
Ionised Alkaline Water	-20 mV to -400 mV

Table 2: The ORP values of different foods. Measured by Dr Dina Aschbach

Chapter 4: Oxidative stress – the energy thief

Every living being needs energy to live. Plants receive their energy from sunlight and generate chemical energy. This is the foundation for the production of bioelectric energy and enables animal and human life. The impacts of civilization cause that energy is "stolen" from humans and animals by destroying the bioelectric energy through oxidation: The so-called "oxidative stress" arises.

Formation and action of secondary free radicals

The term "oxidative stress" means a burden mostly caused by our technical civilization, which is considered to be the (co-)cause of most lifestyle diseases.

This stress is generated by the secondary free radicals, oxidizing agents based on oxygen, also called reactive oxygen species ROS.

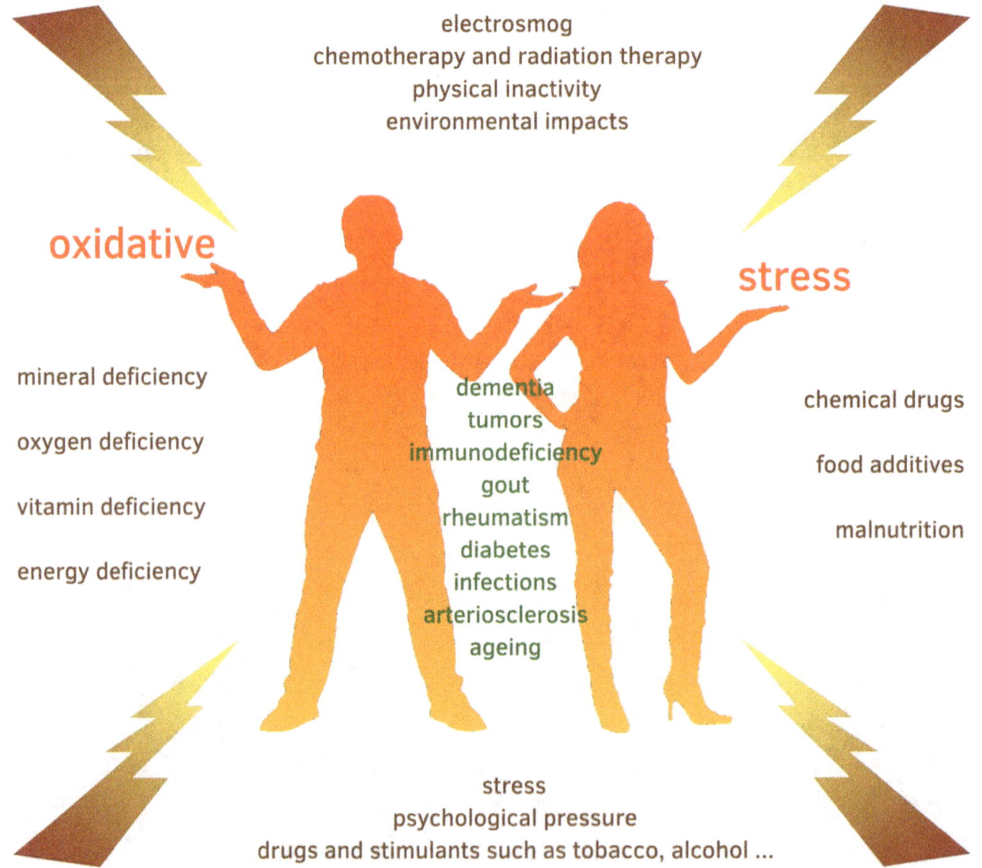

Fig. 24: Oxidative stress – causes and effect

There are different forms of free radicals (these are marked with a · in the chemical formula notation):

- The **hyper oxide anion or superoxide $O_2^-\cdot$** is formed in the energy production process in the mitochondria and is also caused by wrong breathing. It is the most common radical in humans. It is very reactive and can thus damage cell structures. The superoxide is primarily degraded by an enzyme called superoxide dismutase, which converts the radical into hydrogen peroxide H_2O_2 with the help of hydrogen - the further degradation to water and oxygen is done by another enzyme called catalase.

- The **hydroxyl radical HO·** is the most common radical in the atmosphere and is structured like an OH⁻ ion, but missing one electron. It is formed in the atmosphere from ozone O_3 and water vapour under the influence of UV rays. In the body, hydroxyl radicals are formed by ionising radiation, heavy metal molecules and so on, "shooting out" electrons from OH⁻-compounds. The **Perhydroxyl radical HOO·** is formed in a similar way.

- The **Peroxyl radical ROO·** is also formed by oxidation (R is a "residue", an organic molecule). The **Alkoxyl radical RO·** results from the oxidation of fats.

Other molecules that are not directly free radicals but act similarly are:

- **H_2O_2 hydrogen peroxide**, a very strong oxidizing agent, which is formed during the metabolism of sugar molecules.

- **ROOH hydro peroxide**, also a very strong oxidizing agent, which is produced by the modification of organic molecules like fats by ionising radiation, heavy metals and so on.

- **O_3 ozone**, a gas that is produced in the air by pollution and has a strong oxidizing effect on the organism. It splits into oxygen O_2 and a so-called

- **Singlet oxygen O**, which is also very aggressive and wants to oxidize other molecules.

On the one hand, these secondary free radicals form endogenously in the cells during the combustion or oxidation of sugars and fats in the mitochondria. The better the combustion / oxidation process, the fewer free radicals are formed. For a good and complete oxidation, a balanced ratio of oxygen and sugar is necessary as well as an undisturbed oxidation process. Disturbing factors are, for example, over-acidified connective tissues around the cell, which hinders oxygen transport, or chemical substances which hinder oxidation.

On the other hand, free radicals can also be formed exogenously – by external influences –, above all by ionising or radioactive radiation and by oxidising substances such as cigarette smoke and other pollutants.

Free radicals especially like to attack proteins and other protein- and fat-containing molecules in the body and oxidize them, since these molecules are very complex and can easily surrender electrons. DNA (deoxyribonucleic acid, genetic material) is also an easy victim, as are the proteins in the membranes of body cells, enzymes and other molecules that are important for life. Fats and proteins change their properties through oxidation and can even have a damaging effect. If they are irreparably damaged, they must be eliminated by the body or disposed of in "depots" where they can cause diseases such as arteriosclerosis.

By damaging proteins and fats, free radicals are triggers of most diverse ailments and diseases, in particular in combination with over-acidification, because similar to rust being enhanced by acids, proteins weakened by oxidative stress are especially fast attacked by acids and destroyed and/or denatured. Free radicals can thus be regarded as "precursors" for most civilization and lifestyle diseases – sufficient antioxidants are thus the best precaution against these diseases and the prerequisite for a functioning immune system.

Electrons are volatile

Humans and mammals are unable to store free electrons. Antioxidants or free electrons for neutralizing free radicals must therefore be continuously produced or supplied in order to prevent oxidative stress.

Unlike humans and mammals, plants can store the electrons they absorb from photons from sunlight. Plants store electrons mainly in their fruits or seeds in electron-rich antioxidant molecules, protecting the growing germ from oxidation. However, this storage is limited in time. As soon as a plant dies or the fruit or seed is picked or falls off, a creeping "discharge" begins. When all free electrons are discharged, putrefactive bacteria, fungi etc. can "attack" the fruit and the decomposing and rotting process begins.

This shows the difference between animals and plants: after death, meat begins to decompose and rot within a few hours without preservation and uncooled, while an organically grown apple is still "crisp" or at least intact after several months, even without a protective wax layer.

The cultivation method of fruit and vegetables also has an influence on the antioxidant content: apples treated with fertilisers, herbicides and pesticides have considerably fewer antioxidants or lose them more quickly, so they rot faster and therefore need to be treated with anti-fouling agents, while organically grown apples, which dry up and shrivel over time, are still edible and provide a good fertilisation or growth environment for a sprouting apple kernel.

In the food industry, the so-called **ORAC value** (ORAC = Oxygen Radial Absorbance Capacity) is becoming increasingly important. It is intended to show how many effective free electrons a nutrient has with which it can neutralise free oxygen radicals and thus have an antioxidant effect. Organically grown food usually has a higher ORAC value than conventional food.

Antioxidants and Ageing

The apple example shows that antioxidants have an influence on the ageing process of plants.

In mammals, the exact biological cause of the ageing process is still disputed in science. There is much evidence to suggest that ageing is mainly determined by the ability of the body's cells to divide. In contrast to stem cells, which can divide indefinitely, "functional cells" divide about 70 times and then die. This phenomenon can be explained by the **telomere theory**, which states that the end sections of the chromosomes in the cell, the so-called telomeres, become shorter with each cell division – like a lizard sheds its tail, each chromosome thus loses a small end section during cell division. It was later discovered that free radicals and the resulting oxidative stress accelerate the shortening of telomeres. Therefore, if we want to reach our biologically possible age, we have to make sure that the telomeres are not shortened prematurely by free radicals.

Antioxidants against oxidative stress

The redox potential (ORP), describing the excess or lack of free electrons in our body, is difficult to measure, because although electrons are formally always "assigned" to a molecule, in reality they only have a "probability density", which means that – depending on the surrounding molecules – there are more or less electrons in a certain space, and furthermore also in different concentrations. If a measurement is now made in living tissue, the balance of electrons is disturbed, causing a "shifting" of the electrons and influencing the measured values.

Comparatively easy is measuring the ORP in the blood. It can be determined that the ORP in healthy arterial blood is approx. -57 mV, in venous blood approx. -7 mV, both in the slightly negative range with a more or less high surplus of electrons. The redox potential in tissues and organs is in this range as well. All foods and beverages with a higher redox potential henceforth "steal" electrons from the tissue, reducing its energy and making it susceptible to free radicals – these are almost all processed foods and beverages.

The "opponents" of free radicals are antioxidants, electron donating molecules able to neutralize free radicals with excess electrons. The best-known antioxidant is vitamin C – a vitamin C iron solution has a redox potential of -20 mV. Other important antioxidants include vitamin E, glutathione, coenzyme Q10, magnesium, zinc, etc.

The task of antioxidants is it thus to intercept the continuous "attacks" of the free radicals and to prevent cell damage and diseases. The work of the antioxidants can be supported by the supply of free electrons, e.g. from electron-rich drinking water, which recharges them again and again, increasing their lifespan and effectiveness and preventing them from becoming oxidizing agents themselves. *(See Tab. 2, page 27)*

Electrosmog – more than just an electron robber

The increasing, permanent and often continuous presence of electromagnetic radiation (microwave radiation, electrosmog) has profound effects on the electron structure not only in our body, but also in nature, in plants and animals.

Radiations from mobile phones, Wi-Fi and other devices are very strong robbers of electrons and thus one of the biological causes of "civilization-induced" free radicals and oxidative stress, affecting all living beings.

In our body, microwave radiation unfolds a very intensive effect which is further increased by heavy metals such as lead or mercury, for example from amalgam fillings. The heavy metal atoms, which like to be deposited in organs and in the brain, act as small antennas, picking up and amplifying the microwave signals. But also, the water molecules themselves are good antennas, which can be excited and irritated by these external microwaves.

Microwave radiation increases the free radicals in our body both directly, by "shooting" electrons out of the molecules, and indirectly. An indirect effect of the increase of free radicals in the body by microwave radiation, for example, is the obstruction of the formation of the hormone **melatonin** in the pineal gland – a gland in the centre of our brain. Melatonin not only ensures a good night's sleep, but is also a powerful antioxidant, a radical scavenger, therefore, its deficiency increases the formation of free radicals in the body. This is why electrosmog is the cause of massive sleep disturbances. Wi-Fi, cordless and mobile phones should be switched off overnight and the sleeping place should be shielded against radiation from outside.

The excitation of the water molecules by microwave radiation occurs not only in our body, but also in nature and especially in the atmosphere, where the water molecules are omnipresent as water vapour and humidity. We can heat and boil water in a microwave oven because the oscillation movement of the water molecules is stimulated just as strongly by the microwave radiation as by the supply of heat. The same process takes place in the atmosphere: The omni-present microwave radiation causes all water molecules in the air to oscillate at an increased speed. This makes the formation of water clusters and droplets more difficult, the water molecules rise into ever higher layers of the atmosphere. In recent decades, the water vapour content of the upper atmospheric layers has increased significantly – in the stratosphere, the particularly sensitive layer between 15 and 50 km above sea level, the increase over the last 50 years has been more than 75%. The water vapour content was measured by commercial aircraft equipped with sensitive measuring instruments. Water vapour is at least as dangerous a "climate gas" as the much-criticised CO_2, because water vapour also influences the solar radiation and heat radiation of the earth - only water vapour cannot be "taxed" like CO_2.

Chapter 5: Acid and alkaline – the pH value

The contrast of acid and alkaline is the second essential reaction mechanism, maintaining life through the suspense between two poles and enabling reactions of the substances in our body. By definition, acids have a pH value between pH 0 (very strongly acidic) and pH 6.9, bases between pH 14 (very strongly alkaline) and pH 7.1 - pH 7 is neutral.

All substances that can release protons are called acids.

All substances that can absorb protons are called bases.

Moody pH

In German, someone who is angry about something says "I am acidly", meaning "I am angry" or "I am annoyed". Anyone who has ever been really angry knows that the body reacts: Breathing goes faster, the pulse goes up, the muscles are tense – the "mood" is transferred to the body and influences the physical body functions and conditions.

Your mood is	angry/annoyed/"acidic"	in balance
Breathing	fast	Slow
Blood pressure	high	Normal
Pulse	increased	balanced
Heart rates	rigid	Variable
Nervous system	restless	balanced
Muscles	tense	Relaxed
Blood sugar	elevated and volatile	Even

Table 3: The body's reaction on moods

Formation of acids and bases

In pure water, the reaction of water molecules H_2O with each other splits approximately every $10,000,000^{th}$ (10^{7th}) H_2O molecule into H^+ and OH^-. This is called the **natural dissociation** of water. With 10^{-7} H^+ or OH^- ions each, the ratio between these two is in equilibrium and the water is neutral.

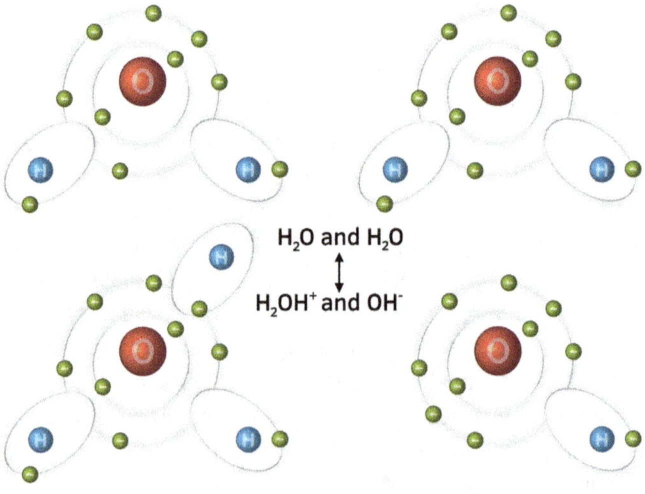

This value can be influenced either by adding acidic substances to the water, which increase the concentration of H^+ ions – also written H_2OH^+ or H_3O^+ – the pH goes down, or by adding alkaline substances to the water, which reduce the concentration of H^+ ions – the pH goes up.

Fig. 25: The natural dissociation of water

In chemistry, the hydrogen ion concentration is indicated by the pH value.

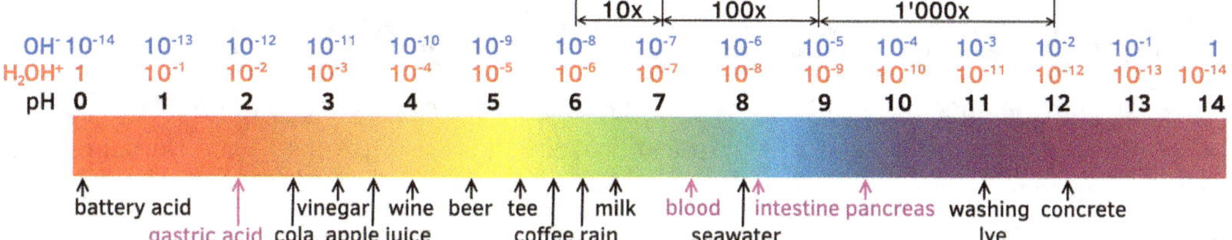

Fig. 26: pH-values (black) and the corresponding amounts of OH⁻ - (blue) and H₂OH⁺ (red) – ions plus the pH values of different liquids. 1 pH equals to 10 times the concentration

The pH value is the negative decadic logarithm of the hydrogen ion concentration:

$$pH = 1 /\log[H^+] = -\log[H^+]$$

Since the concentration values are given logarithmically, a leap from pH 3 to pH 2, for example, means a tenfold increase in the acid concentration, or a leap from pH 7 to pH 9 a hundredfold increase in the base concentration.

Acids have a high concentration of H^+ ions (hydrogen ions which lack one electron). Often, but not always, acids are therefore oxidizing.

Bases, on the other hand, have a high proportion of OH^- ions (hydroxyl ions), which have at least one excess electron. Often, but not always, bases can therefore have a reducing effect.

The approximate pH value can be measured very easily by means of indicators. These are chemicals which change colour according to the change in ph. Known indicators include litmus (acidic: red, alkaline: violet) and thymol blue (strongly acidic: red, acidic to neutral: yellow, alkaline: blue). Mixtures of different indicators can cover the entire pH range by a gradual colour change from red to yellow, green, blue and violet. Red cabbage juice, for example, is a natural indicator that is red in the slightly acidic range, blue in the alkaline range and turns green and yellow at even higher pH values. Electronic measuring instruments are more accurate.

Sour does not always act acidic

Whether a substance acts acidic or alkaline in the body is quite independent of its taste. Many extremely sour beverages, such as lemon juice, consist mainly of organic acids which are converted to carbon dioxide by combustion in the body's cells and excreted through the lungs. This way of de-acidification is still working well in most people. The human body is designed to excrete large amounts of carbon dioxide, and therefore most organic acids do not cause problems.

The effect of substances in the body primarily depends on the elements that are not metabolized in the body to carbon dioxide and excreted through the lungs or otherwise leave the body as gas. These substances are primarily the minerals that remain as ashes when food is burned.

Thus, vegetables and fruits contain an excess of alkaline minerals and have an alkaline effect on the body. Meat, for example, contains an excess of acidic minerals and thus has an acidic effect.

Especially problematic are manmade acidic substances which do not occur in nature. For these substances, such as the orthophosphoric acid – an artificial form of phosphoric acid contained in Coke –, the body has not developed excretion mechanisms. Thus, these substances are very difficult for the body to excrete, they must be concentrated, neutralized with the body's own bases, solidified and deposited somewhere in the body. The same applies to all the other synthetic substances, which are added as nutritional additives to industrially produced foodstuffs, dissolved as traces from plastic containers – like PET bottles – or coated vessels – like Teflon pans – or absorbed by contaminated foods or water: They are very difficult to excrete.

Chapter 6: Hyperacidity, a lifestyle disease

The acid-base balance substantially determines the basic chemical regulation of the human body. Conscientiously it regulates respiration, circulation, digestion, excretion, immune system, hormone balance and so on.

Our body contains about one hundred billion cells. In each of these cells, hundreds of mitochondria (cell bodies) continuously produce energy, carbon dioxide CO_2, water and acidic metabolic residues. Carbon dioxide forms carbonic acid in water and is thus transported to the lungs and excreted. The cell metabolism constantly produces uric acid, which can be excreted by the kidneys. Thus, all energy-producing processes in the organism are acid-forming.

Further acids are formed by acidic minerals in the food. Depending on the minerals contained in the food, the corresponding acid is formed, like phosphoric and sulphuric acid from meat, phosphoric acid from the orthophosphoric acid in cola drinks, which is very difficult to degrade, and so on. Furthermore, other acids are formed in the intestines as a result of rotting processes: hydrogen sulphide, ammonia, histamines, indoles, phenols and skatole are regarded as the cause of skin diseases, allergic reactions and liver damage. Indoles are even classified as carcinogenic.

Today, a **blood serum** with a pH value of around pH 7.4 ± 0.05 is regarded as normal. If the pH value rises above 7.45, it is called alkalosis, if it falls below pH 7.35, it is called acidosis. It is interesting to note that in older medical books the average blood pH value is stated as pH 7.3 – and that today blood pH values far exceed pH 7.5! in people suffering from lifestyle diseases like diabetes, cancer and so on. Their blood therefore contains a multiple of bases compared to a pH value of pH 7.3 previously classified as "average".

Now you may think: "Alkaline blood is good" – but unfortunately this is not the case. The body actively transports the substances it needs via the bloodstream – an excess of alkaline substances in the blood is a reaction of the body to over-acidified connective tissues and a kind of "rescue operation". The body reacts to the "warning messages" of the cells, which, due to the hyper-acidified connective tissue, are neither sufficiently supplied with nutrients and oxygen nor properly cleaned of acid waste. The alkaline substances required for this rescue operation are taken from the body's base depots (hair, bones) – with known consequences such as osteoporosis, hair loss, and so on.

Buffer in our body

Many sophisticated mechanisms help to stabilize the pH value of the blood serum. Substances stabilizing pH value are called buffers. Buffers have the ability to bind ions and remove them from solutions if their concentration becomes too high. On the other hand, buffers can also release ions if their concentration in a solution becomes too low. Buffers thus prevent the pH value from fluctuating too much. This is a very important function, since many biochemical reactions in living organisms release or require ions, but can only take place in a very narrow pH range.

The buffers in the blood cause us not to drop dead immediately after drinking a glass of cola, for example – because theoretically a glass of cola with pH 2.5 would lower the pH value of 10 litres of slightly alkaline body fluid with pH 7.2 to approx. pH 3.6 with the result that the protein in the body would coagulate abruptly and we would be dead on the spot! The pH values of our body fluids range from pH 2.5 (gastric acid) to pH 9 (pancreas).

Hyperacidity is located in the lymph

Since oxidation (combustion) always produces acids in the cells (even with an alkaline diet, the metabolic processes produce more acids than bases), the body always excretes acids. The acids are transported out of the cells through the lymph fluid and excreted:

Carbon dioxide CO_2 and other gaseous acids are excreted via blood and respiration, uric acid and other liquid acids as urine via the kidneys and various other acids as sweat via the skin. If the excretion capacity is exhausted, the pH value of the lymph slowly decreases.

If the lymph becomes acidic, its protein structures harden and it becomes gel-like, viscous and inert. However, an acidic, gel-like and viscous lymph can no longer sufficiently fulfil its function as a transport system and the supply and disposal of cells suffer from its consistency: On the one hand, the cells no longer receive sufficient oxygen and nutrients; on the other hand, acid residues (slags) can no longer be removed from the combustion processes taking place in the cells.

This means for example that **high blood pressure** occurs when the body reacts to the lack of oxygen in the cells caused by the poor transport performance of the over-acidified lymph. Our body regulation increases the blood pressure in order to press more oxygen into the lymph to improve the oxygen supply of the body cells.

The development of **diabetes** can also be understood in this way: The body reacts with raising the blood sugar level to the sugar deficiency in the cells, which occurs when the sugar is prevented from reaching the cell by the hyper-acidified lymph.

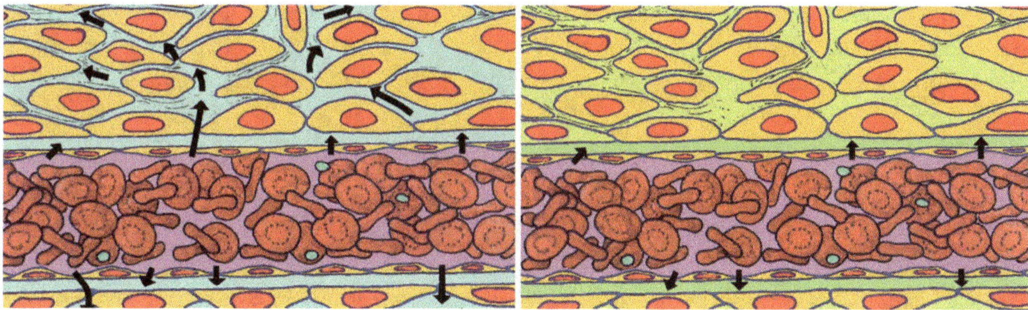

Fig. 27: Transport of nutrients and oxygen from a blood capillary to the body cells in alkaline (left) and acidic (right) lymph fluid

The approximate pH value of the lymph can be easily determined with the pH value of **fresh saliva**. The saliva pH value is meaningful if it is measured after at least two hours without eating and drinking. It should be slightly alkaline, around pH 7.2. Many textbooks state that an acidic saliva pH value is normal, however, this only shows that most people are over-acidified, not that the acidic saliva pH value is healthy – healthy teeth can only remain healthy for a long time in a slightly alkaline environment. The saliva pH value says a lot about the acid-base balance and only changes slowly. With a saliva pH of 7 to 6 we are slightly, under pH 6 chronically over-acidified. In severe diseases like cancer, we find a saliva pH values below pH 6.

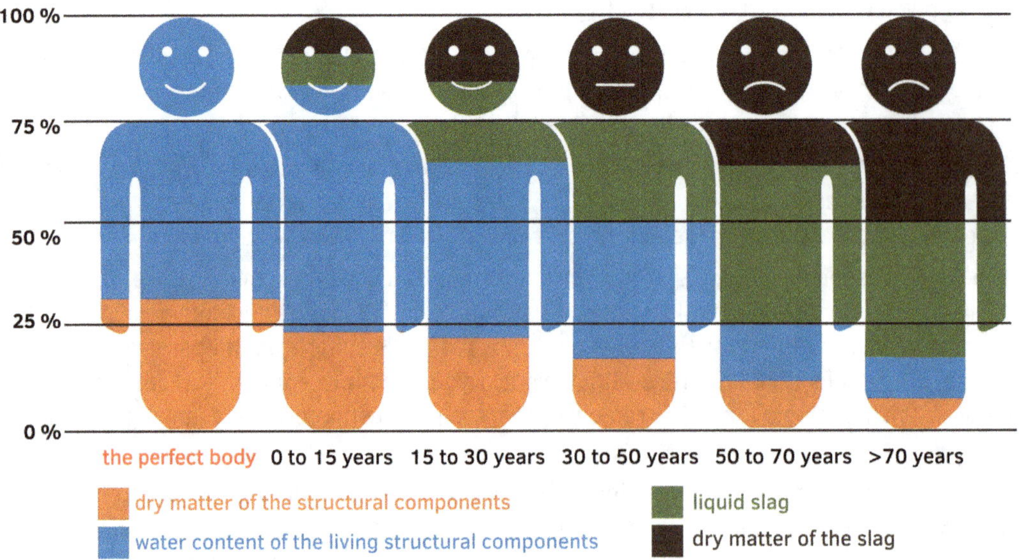

Fig. 28: The slagging of the body increases with age

To alleviate the hyperacidity of the lymph and to prevent a life-threatening hyperacidity of the connective tissues, the body uses a trick: it concentrates, binds and consolidates the excess acids with alkaline minerals, such as calcium from the bones, and deposits these salts for example as calcium sulphate (a salt from calcium and sulphuric acid). These salts form acidic slags as kidney stones, rheumatic deposits on the joints and in the connective tissues, deposits in the blood vessels or they are simply concentrated in the connective tissues in liquid form in one place.

Local acid concentrations cause local blood coagulation, so that especially thin capillaries and peripheral organs are less well supplied with blood. Often acids are deposited as fatty tissues (fatty acids) in the sub cutis and between the organs and thus prevent sufficient blood flow to the adjacent organs.

The places of acid deposition and the order of emptying the base depots seem to be genetically predisposed and hereditary.

For example, in families with an increased risk of diabetes, the excess acids are predominantly deposited in the abdominal cavity next to the pancreas in the form of acid salts or acid salt solutions. This hinders the blood circulation and the supply of the pancreas and leads to dysfunctions with the known consequences.

In families with an increased risk of heart attack or stroke, the acid depots are mainly formed in the arteries, in families with frequent occurrence of rheumatic diseases like gout, arthrosis, arthritis, etc. in the joints. Also inherited receding hairline and hereditary hair loss only indicate that the bodies in this family, for genetic reasons, use the mineral depots of the hair root first, before they resort to other sources.

When dealing with excess acids, there are two types of people. One type concentrates acids very quickly and stores them, they remain relatively slim and do not feel bad, ignoring the "normal" aches and pains, complaints and ailments, until suddenly a severe "accident" such as stroke or heart attack occurs. The healthy looking 50-year-old manager who suddenly drops dead after a stroke or heart attack during a forest run is a sad, but not uncommon example. With them, the dissolution of the deposited acid depots can take quite a long time.

                    Dietmar Ferger • Fountain of Youth Water

The other type first dilutes the excess acids with water and stores them slowly, resulting in weight gain, discomfort and indisposition – they are usually more willing to do something for their health. Their overweight is not only fat, but also stored water, a consistent change in dietary habits towards an alkaline, sugar-free diet can quickly yield positive results.

Talking about "hyperacidity", we always talk about over- or hyperacidity of the lymph and the connective tissues, never about the hyperacidity of the organs, the brain or the blood.

The fairy tale of the protective acid layer of the skin

Conventional skin care products have a low pH value, often even advertised that they protect the acidic protective layer of the skin and are "skin neutral". However, the skin is a very important organ for the excretion of acid metabolic residues (slags). Especially the acids which the kidneys cannot process so well are excreted through the skin.

Again, this is a "trick" of nature, turning something considered harmful in something very useful: The acids accumulating as "waste" protect the skin against bacteria and other microorganisms that can attack the body from outside. This acidic protection is constantly "reproduced" – so we always carry a layer of these acidic slags around us to make us as unappetizing and unattractive as possible for microorganisms.

It is therefore completely pointless and even harmful to classify this protective acid layer as something "worthy of protection". On the contrary, the more intensively we remove it, the better the skin can excrete the acids. Acidic body care prevents the skin from fulfilling its function as an excretory organ and thus promotes internal hyperacidity.

Therefore, it is important to avoid acidic skin care products, shower gels, creams etc. and to use good alkaline skin care products.

An alkaline bath over several hours – a bathing time of 12 hours and longer is beneficial! – is an effective method to eliminate deep-seated acid deposits. However, due to high cardiovascular stress level, this should only be done under medical supervision.

Enzymes and hyperacidity

Enzymes are the most active players in our body. Science knows more than 1,000 different enzymes, but by no means all of them have been researched yet and their mode of action determined. Enzymes enable and accelerate biochemical reactions, without them, our body would not be able to "function". They play a key role in metabolism, both in humans and plants, because enzymes enable and control both the citrate cycle, through which mammals "produce" energy, and the photosynthesis of plants. Our nervous system, the absorption of external stimuli and their transmission to the brain, also functions only through enzymes. They are also involved in the control of the immune system.

Enzymes – their names usually end with the suffix "-ase" – consist of various proteins and often of a "core atom", a metal or mineral such as iron, zinc, copper, selenium, germanium, etc. Thus, many trace elements are essential for the formation of certain enzymes. Since enzymes are always formed when needed and then destroyed, their components must always be "in stock" and supplied to the body. However, especially rare substances such as zinc, germanium, molybdenum, selenium and others are no longer contained in modern diets. This may cause problems, since our body is dependent on these elements and needs the work of the enzymes formed with them for a proper functioning.

Interestingly, this **mineral deficiency** is well known in animal feed. Good horse feed contains up to 20 different minerals and trace elements, chicken feed contains at least five, while it is still suggested that a "balanced diet" according to one of the various "food pyramids" provides humans with a complete and comprehensive supply of all substances necessary for life.

In a healthy soil, the various substances of the periodic table of the elements should be present – even if only in traces – so that they can be absorbed by plants – also in traces – and thus also be available for humans. Due to the acid rain, which in the last century has washed out especially the alkaline elements from the upper layers of the earth, and the widespread fertilization with NPK "compound fertilizer" (nitrogen, phosphorus, potassium), which has displaced the other minerals from the soil, the necessary trace elements can hardly be found in our arable soils anymore and thus cannot be absorbed by the plants. The lack of these elements leads to an often not diagnosable deficiency of necessary enzymes, resulting in missing, slow or faulty body reactions.

Since enzymes consist mainly of proteins, they are sensitive to acid. In an acidic environment their activity is reduced and impeded or they cannot be formed at all. Therefore, **hyperacidity** is another cause of enzyme deficiency.

For example, allergy sufferers feel the effect of a missing enzymes: the hormone histamine is released when foreign substances have entered the body or injuries have occurred. It plays a central role in the defence against these foreign substances and causes itching, pain and muscle contraction. Once the histamine has done its job, it is "destroyed" and broken down by several enzymes. These enzymes require molybdenum and copper. If they are missing, the enzymes cannot be formed and the degradation does not take place, the histamine continues to work unhindered – with the known unpleasant consequences of an allergy.

Besides this impressive example, enzymes are generally the "tools" of our body. The macrophages ("big eaters"), for example, are the "soldiers" of the immune system, ingesting foreign bacteria, viruses and fungi, but also dead cells and cell debris and other "waste" in the connective tissues. They work with the help of specialized enzymes that break down the ingested substances into their components so that they can either be excreted or reused. Macrophages are also weakened by an acidic environment, hindering the immune system to react properly.

Oxygen and carbon dioxide in respiration

Oxygen has a good reputation. We associate oxygen with life, freshness and health. It is true that oxygen is vital and our body has adjusted to the 21% oxygen content of the air. However, it is also true that oxygen is a lethal oxidizing agent and oxidizes many substances, making them burn, rust or become rancid.

In the lungs, oxygen O_2 is absorbed into the blood in order to be transported by red blood cells, the erythrocytes, into the capillaries and from there diffuse into the connective tissues and to the cells. The erythrocytes themselves do not consume oxygen, they generate the energy required for their metabolism anaerobically by fermentation processes without oxygen.

After releasing the oxygen in the capillaries, the erythrocytes absorb carbon dioxide CO_2 to bring it to the lungs for exhalation. Both O_2 and CO_2 are stored in **haemoglobin**, the red blood pigment. However, the reactions of haemoglobin depend on the pH value of its environment: the more alkaline it is, the better oxygen O_2 is absorbed and the worse it is released, the more acidic it is, the worse oxygen O_2 is absorbed and the better it is released.

Therefore, the haemoglobin needs an ambient pH value of around pH 7.3 to enable oxygen uptake and release in a balanced ratio. This so-called **Bohr Effect** – named after the Danish physiologist *Christian Bohr*, the father of the physicist *Nils Bohr* – has far-reaching consequences if the blood pH value is rising as a reaction to the hyperacidity of the connective tissue:

Dietmar Ferger • Fountain of Youth Water

the oxygen saturation measurement in our blood shows satisfying or even excellent values, but our body cells are still undersupplied with oxygen, because the haemoglobin in the blood absorbs oxygen well, but has difficulties to release it. The higher the blood pH value raises, the less O_2 reaches the cells.

Another result of the Bohr Effect is that the O_2-loaded haemoglobin can absorb less CO_2, since the transport of CO_2 from the connective tissue is hindered and the concentration of CO_2 in the blood also decreases. The decreasing CO_2 content in the blood in turn accelerates the rise in the pH value, since CO_2 dissolved in liquid is acidic and would lower the pH value.

Next time when you measure blood pressure and blood oxygen, ask your doctor whether she or he is aware of these physiological correlations, because a blood oxygen measurement without knowing and including the blood pH value is relatively worthless.

Through specific breathing exercises, which minimize the oxygen supply and increase the carbon dioxide content of the blood, the pH value of the blood can be lowered again to such an extent that oxygen can not only be absorbed but also released again. Breathing exercises with this effect are known and described in many eastern traditions like the Chinese Tai-Chi, the Indian Vedas and so on, scientifically they were developed by the Russian doctor *Konstantin Buteyko*.

Today, the so-called **Frolov breathing training** is the most modern form of this kind of training, with far-reaching positive effects not only in respiratory diseases, but also on general performance and health. This training is based on the observation that the normal breathing of most people in the modern world is a pathological, stress-related hyperventilation. First, one has to learn breathing with the diaphragm, because most people only breathe with the chest. Then one practices to gradually prolong the exhalation time against resistance in one second increments per week. 20 to 30 minutes are practiced daily until an exhalation time of 30 seconds and longer is reached.

Signs of hyperacidity - the disease spiral

In many publications, naturopathic doctors point out that hyperacidity of the lymph and connective tissues has become a widespread disease because in many people, the proper excretion of acids, produced in digestion and cell metabolism, via lung, kidneys and skin is overloaded.

In German, one says "I am acidic", meaning "I am angry" – illustrating that the human body and psyche are mutually dependent.

This, hyperacidity often appears first in the **mental and psychological area** and in behaviour: An "acidic" person is very easily irritated, dissatisfied, impatient, aggressive and unfriendly. Dissatisfaction and aggression cause **stress**, which is itself a strong "acidifier". Mental and psychological stress can be measured in the blood: it is raising the level of free radicals. **This is the beginning of the disease spiral.**

Unfortunately, mental and psychological stress quickly develops into physical stress, often caused by stress-related poor sleep, the resulting fatigue and other **compensatory reactions** such as alcohol consumption, smoking or excessive eating. This is the second level of the disease spiral. These complaints, which are usually regarded as "**normal impairments and disorders of well-being**", sooner or later develop into more serious illnesses requiring treatment. However, since the treatment usually does not start at the cause, which is the hyperacidity, but only with the symptoms, and attempts to alleviate these symptoms with drugs that often produce acid again, the disease spiral quickly reaches the next levels.

The following diseases can be attributed directly or indirectly to hyperacidity. Unfortunately, they are very rarely treated with intensive de-acidification and detoxification:

- Chronic headaches and migraines
- Immunodeficiency
- Periodontitis and caries
- Constant fatigue
- Heartburn and digestive problems
- Back pain and tense neck muscles
- Eczema and autoimmune diseases of the skin such as neurodermatitis
- Asthma and allergies
- Rheumatism and gout
- Arteriosclerosis
- Overweight
- Cellulite, thick legs and riding breeches
- Depressions

These diseases are indications of poorly supplied and disposed of cells and organs, of deposits caused by the neutralization of excess acids, and of mechanisms and processes in the body that no longer function "properly" because they are hindered by the deposits or an excessive acid concentration. In the absence of causal treatment, the disease spiral quickly reaches other levels of diseases that become life-threatening, such as cancer, diabetes, and so on.

Homeopathic doctors attribute the **decreasing effectiveness of homeopathic remedies** in adults to hyperacidity and the resulting impeded or reduced stimulus and information conductivity of the body: at low pH levels, the body lacks electrons that can transmit information - the homeopathic information remain stuck in the "swamp" of electron-eating acids.

Important for parents and educators: children react particularly fast on the effect of diet. A child who has eaten chocolate bread before going to school, first gets a sugar boost, followed by a sugar deficiency and hyper-acidification for the rest of the day or until it gets the next sugar-boost. To require from this child the ability to learn, to concentrate, to sit still and to rest is torture against its nature.

The causes of hyperacidity

The acid excretion capacity of man is adapted to a pre-civilized, electrosmog- and emission-free environment with a scarce, but mineral- and vitamin-rich food supply and a large amount of exercise. Additional acid loads demand additional endeavours from the organs for acid excretion – however, if not supported properly, the acid flood of a "civilized" lifestyle exceeds the excretory capacity.

The main causes are:

The eating habits not meet the requirements of the body. We usually eat too much, too fast, in the wrong order and at the wrong time of day.

The diet has changed. Today, meat and dairy products are major components of our diet. Meat forms sulphuric acids during digestion, milk protein from other sources than from the own mother is very difficult to assimilate for the human organism.

The quality of food has deteriorated. Preservatives and chemical additives, fertilizers and pesticides are highly acidic, the content of minerals and vitamins has decreased extremely in the last decades.

The intestine is damaged. In many people the symbiotic bacteria of the intestinal flora are massively damaged and displaced by acid-loving fungi.

Body care is acidic. So-called "pH-neutral" care products with an acid pH value impede acid excretion through the skin.

Stimulants such as tobacco, alcohol, sweets, coffee etc. are also strong sources of acids.

Non-ionising radiation caused by electrosmog from mobile phones, television and radio stations and the use of microwave ovens as well as **ionising radiation** caused by radioactivity impedes cell functions. This results in a poorer and incomplete oxidation of the sugar and fat molecules and thus a higher acid load.

Heavy metal pollution – like from amalgam fillings and other sources – produces acidifying toxins in the body and creates an environment for acid-forming bacteria.

Vaccines burden babies and small children with foreign substances and overload the excretory organs so that acids can no longer be excreted properly.

The oxygen level in the body decreases by wrong breathing and by staying in closed rooms as well as by bad air in the cities. Inhaled pollutants form acids in the body that are difficult to excrete. Reduced lung function by air pollutants and smoking obstruct the CO_2 exhalation.

Stress, negative attitude to life and mental and psychological burdens are essential and mostly underestimated factors for hyperacidity. People with a positive attitude, a high tolerance threshold, many friends and a fulfilled, happy life can be spared longer from lifestyle diseases and the consequences of hyperacidity despite "dietary sins" and an unhealthy lifestyle, whereas health freaks who are frightened and suspicious, but doing a lot for their health objectively and leading a perfect healthy lifestyle, produce so much acids in their body that their efforts are cancelled out.

Lack of exercise and lack of sleep also promote hyperacidity.

Today, acid-base balance is found almost exclusively in breastfed babies of healthy, non-smoking mothers.

Chapter 7: Social consequences of the lifestyle diseases

The term "lifestyle diseases" covers diseases which pharmaceutically oriented medicine cannot explain, and thus, of course, not heal. From anti-asthmatics to cancer drugs and sleeping pills, the largest share of drug costs is caused by drugs against lifestyle diseases. In 2018, the total spending for healthcare in the United States reached nearly 11,000 USD per capita (plus 3,000 US$ compared to 2010), in UK about 3,200 £ (plus 1,000 £ compared to 2010, in Australia over 7,100 AU$ (plus 1,600 AU$ compared to 2010), in Germany 4,500 € (plus 1,000 € compared to 2010), and in India about 5,000 ₹ (plus 3,000 ₹ compared to 2010). The health expenditures are everywhere in a sharp rise and reaches in the USA 17% of the GDP! (UK: 10%, Australia: 9,3%, Germany 11% and India 3,2%) *(Source: OECD statistics)*

The lifestyle diseases are rising steadily and seemingly unstoppable and relatively unnoticed by the media: Cancer, heart attacks and strokes seem to attack healthy people out of the blue and rip them out of their lives, often with fatal consequences. The cancer rate in "western" countries is slowly approaching 50%, which means that one in two develops tumours at least once in the course of their lives and is then exposed to the "cancer machinery" of surgery, radiation and chemotherapy – mostly with questionable success and a significant impairment of quality of life.

Diabetes, high blood pressure, osteoporosis, asthma, rheumatism, gout, arteriosclerosis and many other diseases occur rather insidiously, but have a decisive impact on the quality of life, motivation and performance. They make those affected to become regular customers of the medical-industrial complex. Medical doctors, due to a lack of knowledge about the causes of the diseases, tries to alleviate the symptoms with medication and symptomatic treatments, without, however, achieving a real cure. The CDC, the US-American Center for Disease Control and Prevention, headlines on its webpage: "90 % of the nation's $3.3 trillion in annual health care expenditures are for people with chronic and mental health conditions" – whereby "chronic and mental health conditions" are just another word for lifestyle diseases.

While some lifestyle diseases are mainly caused by behaviour like poor nutrition, consumption of sugary and acidic drinks such as cola and soft drinks, lack of exercise and so on, other diseases, especially cancer, seem to be more and more like gambling with a probability of slightly more than 50% not to be among the victims. Like the evil dragon in some fairy tales, cancer claims its victims from our midst, regardless of age, education and gender. In 2016, nearly 300 out of 100,000 in dies of cancer in Germany, 260 of 100,000 in UK, 190 of 100,000 in Australia and USA. *(Source: OECD statistics)* If you take a closer look, however, you will find a cause for every cancer "victim": Microwave radiation from cell phones is among the most common causes, but also stress at the workplace or in the family, air pollution by chemicals or dust, drinking water pollution and so on.

On May 30th, 2018, Reuters made an alarming report. It said:

"China has overtaken the United States in healthy life expectancy at birth for the first time, according to World Health Organization data.

Chinese new-borns can look forward to 68.7 years of healthy life ahead of them, compared with 68.5 years for American babies, the data – which relates to 2016 – showed.

American new-borns can still expect to live longer overall – 78.5 years compared to China's 76.4 – but the last 10 years of American lives are not expected to be healthy."

To get an idea how the disease rate develops, comparing the total life expectancy with the healthy life expectancy is a good tool. The difference between these two lifespans is the sick life time, one depends on medication and cannot live without help. This can serve as an indicator of the health of the life style as well as the quality of the health system in the respective country.

There, for example, we can see that an average Singaporean lives almost eight years longer in good health than the average US citizen. The latter, therefore, is more than three years longer sick than his Singaporean counterpart, whereas in Singapore, the sick life time is even decreasing – in contrast to the development in most other countries, where the sick life time increases continuously.

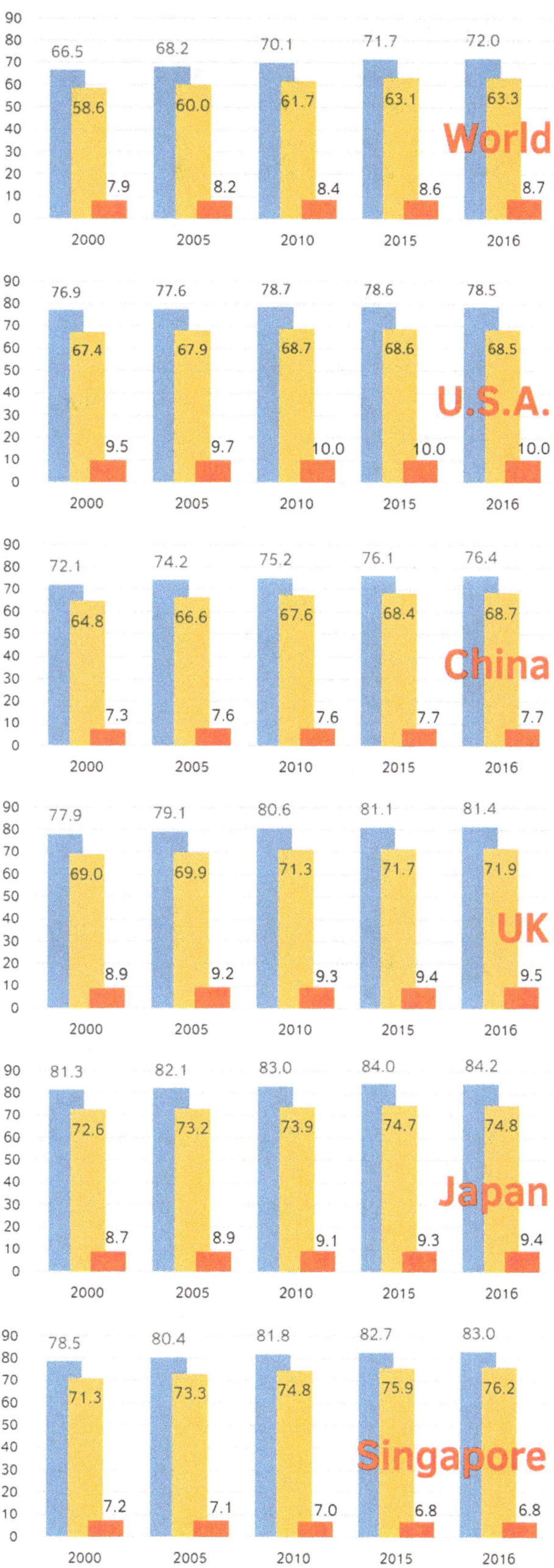

Fig. 29: Life expectancy (blue), healthy life expectancy (yellow) and sick life (red) development in years in the world and in selected countries in order of the healthy life expectancy (Source: WHO)

The costs of the most important lifestyle diseases in US 2015

Circulatory and cardiovascular diseases: $392 billion
       thereof heart conditions: $220 billion
       thereof hypertension: $79 billion

Musculoskeletal diseases: $366 billion
       thereof osteoarthritis: $143 billion
       thereof back problems: $97 billion

Respiratory diseases: $267 billion
       thereof COPD and asthma: $182 billion

Metabolic diseases: $254 billion
       thereof diabetes: $133 billion

Nervous and sense organs diseases: $241 billion

Cancer: $200 billion

Gastrointestinal diseases: $178 billion

Blood diseases: $40 billion

Infectious diseases: $135 billion

Injuries and poisoning: $201 billion

Mental illness: $165 billion

Others: $855 billion

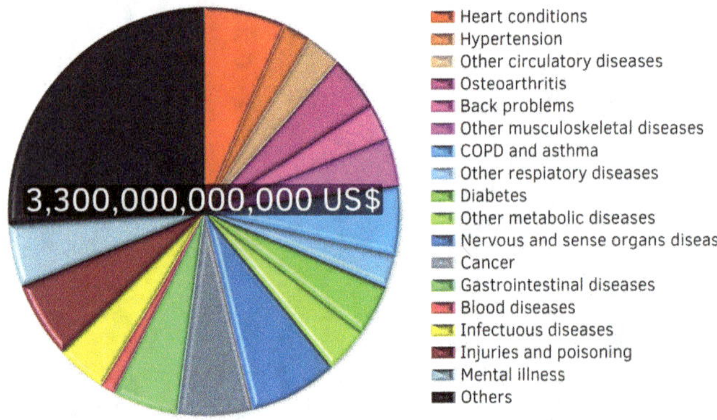

Fig. 30: Proportion of various diseases in the total health care costs in the USA in 2015 (Source: U.S. Bureau of Economic Analysis)

Lifestyle diseases with the highest death toll

Unfortunately, lifestyle diseases do not only impair the quality of life, but are also increasingly the cause of premature death, often preceded by a long ordeal of pain, hospitalisation and the medication with many side effects.

Respiratory diseases, especially COPD and asthma, are the third most common cause of death in the US. According to CDC, 1 of 13 US Americans has asthma, 7.7% of the adults, 8.4% of the children, more than 25 Million people. In 2017, 154,596 people died of respiratory diseases.

Asthma is caused by allergic reactions of the body to substances from the environment, it is a wrong response of the immune system, caused mainly by malfunctions of enzymes. Enzymes are strongly impaired in their effectiveness and functionality by hyper-acidification and lack of trace elements. The stress-induced hyperventilation, which occurs in childhood, also contributes to the development of asthma, as the lungs can no longer be properly ventilated and cleaned. Asthma and most other respiratory diseases such as bronchitis, angina pectoris, etc. are preventable if a lifestyle with less stress is cultivated and healthy, slow abdominal breathing is learned and practised.

        Dietmar Ferger • Fountain of Youth Water

Cancer as the second most frequent cause of death can be treated longer and longer by expensive technologies and medicines with treatment costs of many thousand USD per month. In 2018, 1,735,350 new cancer cases occurred in the USA alone, about 600,000 people died from it, which is 186 per 100.000 inhabitants and 21.7 % of all deaths in the US. Almost every second US citizen will suffer this fate in the course of his life. In 2018, about 18 Million cancer patients have been counted worldwide. Treatment costs differ, since in poor countries the modern cancer treatment is unaffordable to most of the patients. Worldwide, the cancer death toll counted nearly 10 Million people.

About 200 billion USD have been spent for cancer treatment in US in 2015 - with moderate success, because over half of cancer patients still die within 5 years after the first appearance of a tumour.

According to studies by the American Environmental Agency, approximately 35% of cancer cases are caused by poor nutrition and 30% by smoking. However, since factors such as microwave radiation and stress are very difficult to detect and to query, it can be assumed that they also account for a high proportion of the increasing incidence of cancer, especially as they increase other stressful factors. Pharmaceutically oriented medicine is still unable to convincingly present the causes of cancer, which is why all conventional treatment approaches fail at the end. As early as 1924 the Nobel Prize winner, physician and biochemist *Otto Heinrich Warburg* stated that *"the cause of cancer is a replacement of oxygen respiration of the cells by fermentation".* The latest findings confirm his research. Fermentation occurs when the cells are no longer sufficiently supplied with oxygen. The main cause of the oxygen deficiency is the hyperacidity of the connective tissues, which prevents the capillary oxygen from reaching the cells. Hyper-acidified connective tissues also prevent the acidic metabolic residues formed in the body cells from being transported away, so that they remain in the cells, become increasingly acidic and finally switch from oxygen respiration to fermentation. Oxidative stress, which attacks and injures cells, supports the formation of cancer cells.

It can only be called scandalous that despite a cure rate of far below 50%, almost every cancer patient in the rich countries of the world has to undergo the ordeal of surgery, radiation and chemotherapy, whereas alternative approaches implementing the scientific findings of *Otto Heinrich Warburg* and other important doctors and scientists such as *Dr Alfons Weber* and *Dr Johanna Budwig*, have no access to official medicine. It seems that the treatment of cancer is too flourishing an industry to be restricted by more effective methods and treatment measures, which are also much cheaper.

The most frequent cause of death are **cardiovascular diseases**, which is an umbrella term for several conditions, including **atherosclerosis, heart disease, heart failure, stroke, heart attack, arrhythmia, and heart valve problems** – which are all direct or indirect consequences of high blood pressure. In US, cardiovascular diseases cause about one third of all deaths, 850,000 in 2016.

According to the American Heart Association, nearly half of all adults in the United States suffer from cardiovascular diseases and high blood pressure. They take drugs rich in side effects to lower the blood pressure, forgetting that body regulation increases blood pressure with the aim of improving the oxygen supply to the body cells. As with asthma and cancer, the insufficient supply of oxygen to the body's cells is the main cause of cardiovascular diseases. Blood circulation problems are further aggravated by two factors: arteries are narrowed by deposits of coagulated proteins and oxidized fats which have been neutralized by the body's own alkaline minerals. This is falsely called calcification. These constrictions can lead to congestion, which then cuts off body cells and organs from the blood supply, the deposits can also break loose and suddenly block arteries and causing stroke. Oxidation and microwave radiation cause the red blood cells to clump together to so-called "money rolls", resulting in viscous consistence and hindering oxygen transport.

Thus, an unfavourable interaction of hyperacidity, wrong breathing and microwave radiation is often the cause of a sudden and unexpected death or lifelong disability.

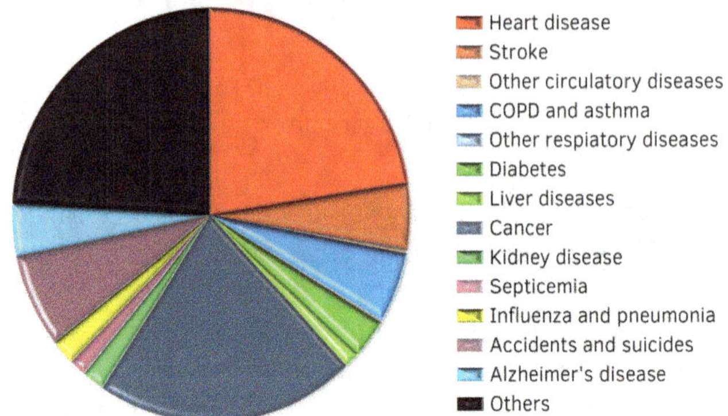

Fig. 31: Causes of death in the US 2017 (Source: CDC)

How we can avoid diseases

The following conclusions can be drawn from these findings about the connections between the chemical and physical processes, taking place in the body to maintain life:

- All life processes take place in **water**. Sufficient water of good quality is therefore a prerequisite for healthy processes in the body.
- Every lifestyle disease (a disease not induced by external influences, bacteria or viruses) is caused by a **disturbance the chemical and physical processes** in the body like the pH value or oxidative stress.
- **Misguided defence mechanisms** of the body to maintain the pH value, to ensure the supply of cells and to fight microorganisms, viruses and so on are also the cause of many diseases. Many diseases can be prevented by supporting and controlling these defence mechanisms.

Long-term health is primarily the result of:

- Supply with sufficient water of good quality
- Supply with all necessary minerals and trace elements
- Neutralization of the oxidative stress caused by civilization
- Maintenance of an alkaline body pH
- Support of the body in the excretion of acid waste products
- Supply with antioxidants.

Chapter 8: Ionised water

21st century medicine is facing two main challenges: On the one hand, exploding numbers of diseases with unknown causes, summarized under the heading "lifestyle diseases". On the other hand, equally explosive numbers of antibiotic-resistant bacteria and fungi which in many hospitals can only be kept in check with the last hard antibiotics – it is only a matter of time before resistance to even these last remedies appear.

Ionised water in its two forms – as hydrogen-rich alkaline ionised water with antioxidant effect and as oxygen-rich acidic ionised water with low pH value and oxidative, disinfecting effect – is a solution for these two problems. Therefore, ionised water is a functional water with effects that are of great importance for our modern society.

Ionised water is created by the intelligent symbiosis of water and electricity, in which electricity = energy is "extracted" from the acidic ionised water then stored in the alkaline ionised water. Alkaline ionised water can be produced naturally by the reaction of metallic aluminium, magnesium or similar elements with water.

Through alkaline ionised water, electrical energy and hydrogen can be transferred to become effective for biological systems such as humans, animals and plants. Water is the best medium to transfer hydrogen and electrical energy directly to biological systems.

Alkaline ionised water is therefore a water that gives energy to biological systems and promotes life, while acidic ionised water draws energy from biological systems and suppresses life.

Studies and reports

Natural healing clinics and practices in Japan have been using alkaline ionised water for the longest time, their first known reports date back to 1985. At that time, water ionisers have been very expensive devices, affordable only for professional use. Findings between 1985 and 1990 at naturopathic Japanese clinics document the following results of treatment with alkaline ionised water:

- Lowering of the blood sugar level and improvement of the HbA1c value in diabetes mellitus.
- Improvement of peripheral blood circulation in diabetic gangrene
- Lowering the uric acid level in gout patients
- Improvement of liver function in hepatitis, cirrhosis and other liver diseases
- Improvement in small intestine ulcers and prevention of recurrence of the disease
- Normalization in case of too high and too low blood pressure
- Lowering the cholesterol level
- Improvement in angina and heart muscle disorders
- Improvement in allergic diseases such as asthma, hypersensitivity, atopic dermatitis and nettle rash.
- Improvements in autoimmune diseases and rheumatism
- Improvement in so-called specific diseases, Behcet's disease, Crohn's disease, Kawasaki's syndrome and colon ulcers
- Improvement in malignant liver cancers, hepatomas and metastatic cancers
- Improvement in case of discomfort, chronic constipation and diarrhoea

- Improvement in children after dehydration due to vomiting and diarrhoea in viral diseases
- Improvements in hyperbilirubinemia in new-borns
- Experiences of pregnant women who drank alkaline ionised water during pregnancy: almost no morning vomiting, uncomplicated birth, little jaundice …

Since the first studies in Japan, alkaline ionised water has established itself worldwide – but clinical studies meeting the standards of Western science are rare. This is mainly due to the immense costs of a professional western study design, which can only be paid by pharmaceutical or medical technology companies (and later refinanced by selling the drugs or devices).

For an up-to-date overview of studies, reviews and reports on the effects of ionised water, please visit **www.fountain-of-youth-water.com**.

Alkaline and acidic ionised water are functional waters

Therefore, it would be a great merit for the health care systems in the western countries to document the effectiveness of hydrogen, alkaline and acidic ionised water by means of professional studies and to catalogue and evaluate the many personal reports of experience which are available up to now. These are tasks that should be in the public interest.

We do not want to discuss further the entanglements in the public health care systems, but rather appeal to the reason, the ability to think logically and the chemical-physical-biological knowledge of each individual to take their health into their own hands. This book is meant to be a contribution to strengthen this ability. The right water is certainly an important element of holistic health care. Therefore, hydrogen water or alkaline ionised water are the first choice, even if and precisely because – as critics like to notice – they are not natural waters, but functional waters produced electrically or by contact with magnesium with the function of neutralizing oxidative stress caused by civilization. No more, but also no less. And since oxidative stress, as shown on the previous pages, is the main cause of civilization diseases, hydrogen water and alkaline ionised water can play an important role.

On the other hand, to combat the increasingly resistant germs and bacteria, acidic ionised water is the best solution, because it is a functional water at least equal to modern disinfectants in most cases, but free of side effects, inexpensive and without resistance formation. Particularly in the case of globally rampant infections such as the corona virus, this technology should also be used worldwide – because unlike chemical disinfection, it has no harmful effects on nature.

Chapter 9: The history of water ionisation

Development in Japan and Korea

Initial research into the use of alkaline ionised water in agriculture and livestock breeding began in Japan in 1931, when researcher *Machisue Suwa* began to investigate the relationship between electricity and water. He experimented with many different types of water and in 1952 developed the first water electrolysis device capable of producing alkaline and acidic ionised water. At that time, the alkaline ionised water was called *"Synnohl liquid"*.

In 1954, the first industrial water ioniser for use in agriculture was developed in cooperation with the University of Tokyo and subsequently its use was studied by various agricultural universities, especially in rice cultivation. It was found, for example, that rice grains germinated in alkaline ionised water sprout faster, produce higher yields and require less water. This was called the *"Synnohl agricultural method"*. These units consisted of two water-filled chambers in which electrolysis plates were hung, separated by a membrane.

Driven by cooperation with the University of Tokyo and clinical research conducted there, as well as by reports from users who drank the water produced by the agricultural devices, the first water ioniser for household use was launched in 1958, and in 1960 the first medical research institute for researching alkaline active water and its effects was founded, the *"Synnohl Liquid Medical Science Research Association"*, whose work shifted the focus of water research more towards the medical field. In 1962, alkaline ionised active water was officially classified as medically effective by the Japanese Ministry of Health. Water ionisers were developed by various companies and came onto the market.

The classification of ionised water as medically effective substance referred to the following indications:

- Alkaline ionised water: Drinking is effective against chronic diarrhoea, indigestion, stomach and intestinal complaints, acidic burping and heartburn.

- Acidic ionised water: For external use as anti-inflammatory agent and for personal hygiene and beauty

When the first direct flow water ioniser came onto the market in 1979, it was referred to as "alkaline ionised water" and "acidic ionised water" in as it is commonly used today. Due to the growing interest in health and water quality and the easier handling of the devices, they became more and more popular until 1992, when a health programme on Japanese television, in which the "miracle water" was presented, made the breakthrough. This media attention also increased the need for further research, so that in 1993 a university research project was launched to prove the safety and effectiveness of alkaline ionised water beyond any doubt. In 1997, the positive effect on gastrointestinal complaints was officially confirmed as proven, and in 1999 the project was completed with the result that alkaline ionised water is useful and safe and that the indications certified in 1962 could be confirmed. Together with the Association of Water Ioniser Manufacturers founded in 1992 and based on this research, specifications and standards for household water ionisers were drawn up and made mandatory in Japan.

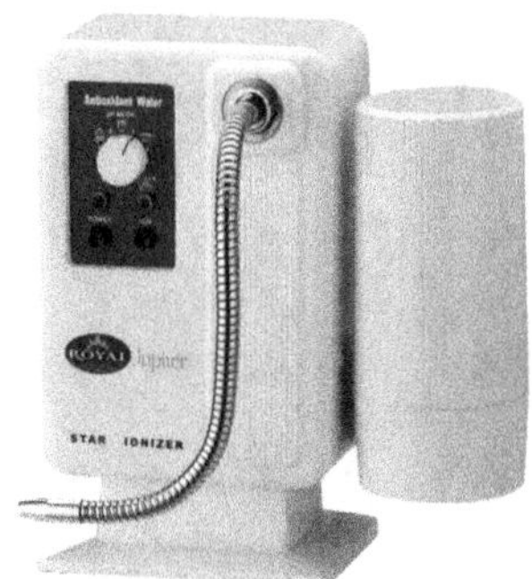

Fig. 32: The first Japanese direct flow water ioniser

In the meantime, the first water ionisers were built according to Japanese standards in Korea, at that time mainly an "extended workbench" of Japan. Since 2000, production in Japan and Korea, has increased considerably, new companies have entered the market and improved design and function. Today, electric water ionisers are also being built in Taiwan and China, mostly following the Japanese design and often with Japanese components. In parallel, materials research at Japanese, Korean and Chinese universities is improving functional bioceramics in such a way that better and better mineral water ionisers are coming onto the market.

In Japan, the Japanese Pharmaceutical Products Law was revised in 2005, in which water ionisers were described as medical devices for domestic use and defined in the medical field as "devices for producing alkaline ionised drinking water to improve gastrointestinal symptoms". In Korea this classification was adopted.

A new chapter in water research began in 2007. *Dr Mitsuhiro Ohta* of Kobe University published a detailed study, proving that the health benefits of alkaline ionised water are mainly due to the presence of hydrogen in gaseous (molecular) form. Since 2007, research has been carried out worldwide into how hydrogen can be used as a medical gas.

Development in the Soviet Union

Around 1970, research on alkaline and acidic ionised water also began in the Soviet Union. **Catholyte** (strong alkaline ionised water) and **anolyte** (strong acidic ionised water) were made from salt solutions and used for technical purposes. In order to improve the physicochemical properties of the flushing liquid used in the borehole during natural gas and oil production in the Uzbek desert and to emulsify the gushing oil, Russian and Uzbek engineers had developed a device for the electrical separation and activation of water enriched with salt, and successfully used the catholyte formed on the alkaline side for this purpose. The acidic anolyte, which is formed at the same time, was used to consolidate the clay and sludge masses.

By chance, an engineer suffering from allergic skin reactions and ulcers – which were very common due to the immense environmental pollution caused by oil production – noticed that contact with the anolyte reduced ulcers and allergic reactions. The workers also noticed that catholyte soothed the sunburn and began to bathe in it to protect themselves against the harmful effects of the hot Uzbek desert sun.

Subsequently, research was intensified. In Tashkent, extensive research with ionised water was carried out funded by the government. The military was interested in the germicidal and disinfectant effect of the anolyte, because in the Soviet Union during the Cold War there was fear of an American attack with bacteriological weapons. It turned out that anolyte was the antidote they were looking for: cheap and easy to produce, highly effective in destroying unicellular organisms such as bacteria, harmless and without side effects for humans and nature.

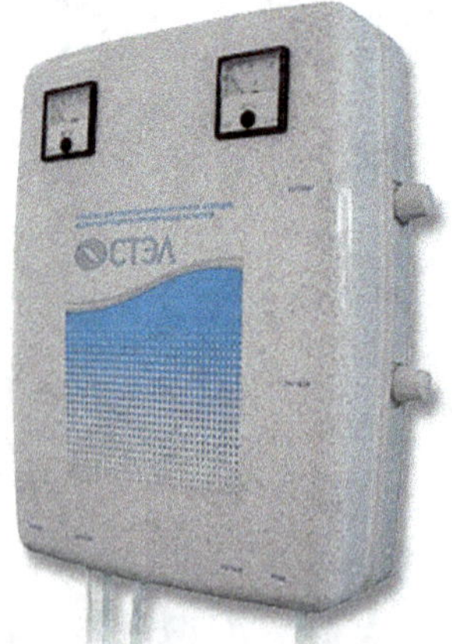

At the same time, the effects of the catholyte on living beings were investigated and it was found that it helped not only against solar but also against ionising radiation and that it is suitable as radiation protection – but these findings were kept secret and disappeared in the archives. After the reactor accident in Chernobyl, catholyte and alkaline ionised water were also used to help radiation-damaged patients.

Fig. 33: Russian device for production of anolyte and catholyte

Dietmar Ferger • Fountain of Youth Water

In addition to medical research, research was also carried out into their use in agriculture, especially in animal breeding, and it was shown that regular administration of diluted anolyte greatly reduces or almost eliminates the use of antibiotics in animal husbandry, while at the same time improving animal health and meat quality.

Until the collapse of the Soviet Union, research on the "**water of life**" (alkaline ionised water, catholyte) and the "**water of death**" (acidic ionised water, anolyte) – as the Russians called the ionised water – was intensively researched. There were several research groups staffed with highly qualified scientists in the most diverse fields of research, especially around the engineer *Vitold Bakhir*, who still heads an institute in Russia today.

Today, in the successor states of the Soviet Union, water ionisation devices are mainly produced for commercial applications, the use of anolyte and catholyte in the food industry and in agriculture is widespread. Anolyte is used as a disinfectant in almost all Russian hospitals.

Development in Germany

Long before research began in Japan, research on electro-activated water was carried out in Germany and products were developed - unfortunately, research and development ended around 1981, knowledge and products are forgotten today.

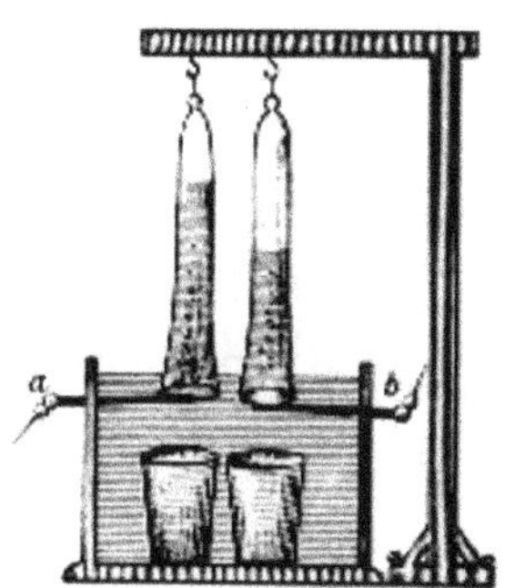

Fig. 34: The first electrolysis device of Johann Wilhelm Ritter

Johann Wilhelm Ritter was a contemporary of *Johann Wolfgang Goethe* and *Wilhelm von Humboldt* and studied in Jena after completing his training as a pharmacist. He devoted himself to the recently discovered electrical energy, researched galvanism and developed the electrochemical theory, which is the knowledge that galvanic and electrical processes are always associated with oxidation and reduction. In 1802, he built the first electrolysis device with which he was able to produce hydrogen and oxygen gas. He was the first to quantitatively determine the ratio between the two gases. He then built the first battery by placing cardboard discs soaked in salt solution between 50 copper plates and electrifying them.

In 1809, *Ferdinand Friedrich Reuss*, a chemist born in Tuebingen and professor at the University of Moscow, showed that water diffuses through clay when a current is applied – the electro-osmotic principle. In 1921, the chemist *Count Botho von Schwerin* applied for a patent for the production of "artificial mineral water" with this principle and founded the "Elektro-Osmose Aktiengesellschaft" (Electro Osmosis Corporation) in Berlin.

In 1931, the engineer and naturopath *Alfons Natterer* in Munich built the first water ioniser with three chambers to use the mineral-poor water, which is formed in the middle chamber, for brewing beer, because the water in Munich contains a lot of limestone and is not suitable for brewing if untreated. Since the breweries were not interested in his water, he researched health applications and successfully sold the alkaline and ionised acidic water in pharmacies under the name *"Hydropuryl"*. His production facilities were destroyed by a bomb attack in 1940, but he rebuilt them after the war in Berchtesgaden and the Upper Palatinate. Until his death in 1981, his "Muenchner Lebenswasser" ("Munich water of life") was widely used in agriculture and medicine. Together with the German-American physician, sailor and inventor *Manfred Curry*, he developed a method with which he could diagnose a disease by feeling the taste of the strongly alkaline Hydropuryl on his tongue - even the BILD newspaper (the most popular German news-paper) dedicated a large article to this method in 1975.

Chapter 10: Electric water ionisers

Today, technical equipment has conquered households. From slicing bread to cooking eggs, technical helpers are omnipresent. Most of them can be replaced by manual work and serve only for convenience and time saving.

Water ionisers are different. Hardly any other household appliance has such a strong influence on lifestyle and health as this appliance. Since the first direct flow water ioniser, which was developed in Japan in 1979, many millions of households, especially in East and Southeast Asia, have purchased and are using a water ioniser. Currently, almost all health-conscious households in Japan and South Korea, and many households in China and Southeast Asia have a water ioniser or similar device for optimizing and ionising water.

What is alkaline ionised water?

Alkaline ionised water is water that has been physically treated in a water ioniser and has outstanding properties:

- It has a high pH value
- It contains gaseous (molecular) hydrogen.
- It has a low redox potential and thus a large electron surplus.
- It has small water clusters and is therefore "more liquid" than normal water.

What is acidic ionised water?

Acidic ionised water is always produced parallel to alkaline ionised water. Acidic oxide water has opposite properties to alkaline ionised water:

- It has a low pH value
- It contains gaseous oxygen
- It has a high redox potential and thus a large electron deficiency.
- Like alkaline ionised water, it has small water clusters.

How does an electric water ioniser work?

An electric water ioniser is connected to the water pipe in the kitchen. In the first step, it contains an activated carbon filter to clean the water of organic pollutants and to remove chlorine, which may harm and destroy the membrane in the ionising unit. Then it ionises the water by incomplete electrolysis. For this, the water flows in a chamber divided by a fine semi-permeable membrane. On each side of the chamber there are titanium electrodes coated with platinum, one is positively, the other negatively charged. This allows galvanic current to flow. It causes the alkaline minerals to migrate to one chamber and the acidic minerals to the other.

Cations are positively charged alkaline ions, they surround the negative electrode and produce cathode water, which is alkaline ionised water, also called catholyte and, by the Russians, water of life. It contains gaseous molecular hydrogen.

Anions are negatively charged acidic ions, they surround the positive electrodes and produce anode water, which is acidic ionised water, also called anolyte and by the Russians water of death. It contains gaseous oxygen and ozone.

At the same time, the water clusters are restructured and re-assembled into the smallest possible units.

Since only conductive, mineral-containing water can be ionised, the filter often contains a layer of calcium, serving also as a buffer for chloride, which would attack the membrane.

Alkaline ionised water flows from the tap on top of the unit, the acidic ionised water from a hose on the bottom. The alkaline ionised water is used for drinking and cooking. The oxidation potential of the acidic ionised water makes it a good agent for washing hands, rinse the mouth in case of inflammation, cleaning food or kitchen utensils and treating small wounds.

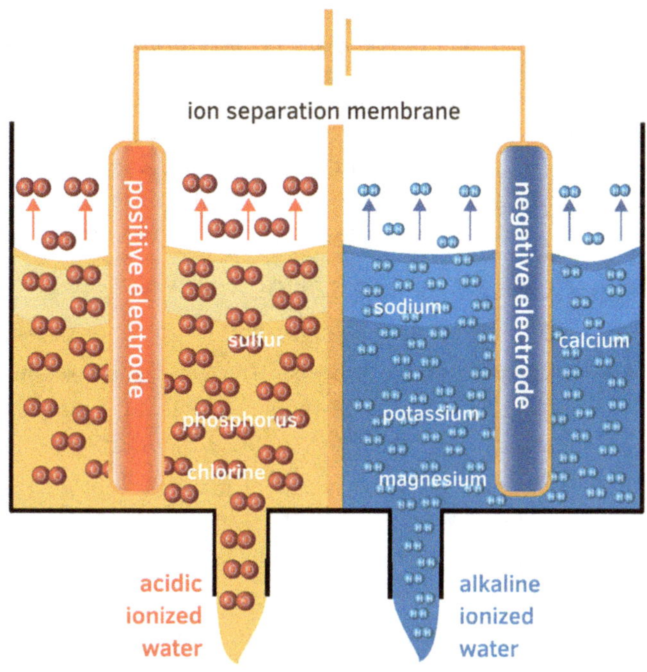

Fig. 35: reactions in an ionisation chamber

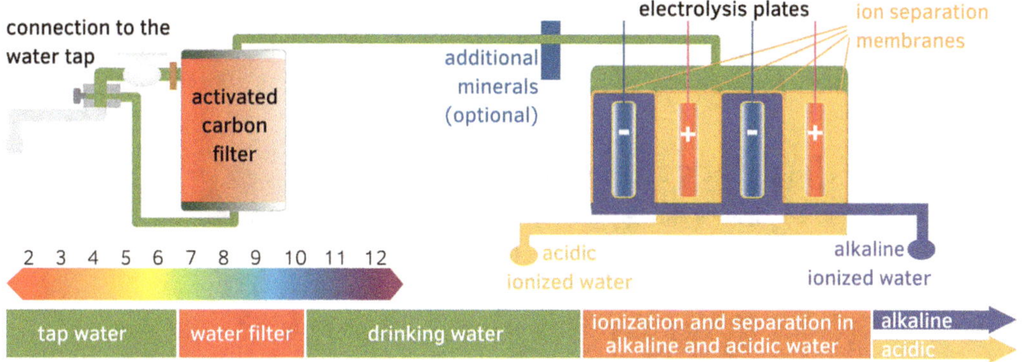

Fig. 36: Flow diagram of a water ioniser with pH scale

Chapter 11: Reactions at the electrodes

Various chemical reactions take place in the ionisation unit of an electric water ioniser. Physically, these reactions are caused by the supply or withdrawal of electrons – electrons are supplied to the water on the cathode side and withdrawn from it on the anode side.
This chapter explains the chemical reaction processes by means of formulas and can be skipped by readers not interested in technical and chemical details.

Prerequisites for ionisation

In order for ionisation to take place, certain conditions must be met. These are:

- A DC voltage at the electrodes. This voltage varies between 12 and 36 volts at the various manufacturers. It must be regulated so that it has maximum effectiveness on the one hand, but on the other hand it must not lead to a short circuit or overheat and damage the control electronics.

- A diaphragm, which is a selectively permeable partition membrane between the electrodes, which is usually made of a special cellulose-based plastic.

- The water must have a certain conductivity, otherwise no current can flow and no ionisation can take place. A conductivity of approximately 50 µS/cm (micro-Siemens per cm) is usually sufficient, which equals a water hardness of about 1.6 °e (English hardness) or 0.12 ppm $CaCO_3$.

The ionisation strength depends on the following parameters:

- The voltage at the electrodes: The higher the voltage, the stronger the ionisation.

- The conductivity of water: the higher the conductivity, the stronger the ionisation.

- The duration of the ionisation: The longer the water remains in the chamber, the stronger the ionisation.

Reactions in the cathode chamber

In the cathode chamber, the negatively charged cathode releases electrons into the water, thus resulting in a strong electron surplus, also called negative charge or negative redox potential. These electrons cause the following reactions, which take place in parallel:

First reaction: The water becomes alkaline:

$$2\,H_2O + 2\,e^- \rightarrow 2\,OH^- + H_2 \uparrow \rightarrow 2\,OH^-$$

In a large surplus of electrons, a hydrogen atom H from a water molecule H_2O is replaced by a free electron, the H_2O becomes a hydroxide ion OH^-. The released hydrogen atom H combines with a second H to form hydrogen gas H_2, which dissolves in the water, which means it "sits" between the water molecules, or it degasses as bubbles.

The excess of OH^--ions makes the water alkaline.

Second reaction: The water receives a negative redox potential,
antioxidant (reducing) and activated (negatively charged) hydrogen is produced:

$$H_2O + 2\,e^- \rightarrow OH^- + H + e^- \rightarrow OH^- + H^-$$

As in the first reaction, the H_2O is converted into OH^-. However, the released hydrogen atom H does not combine with another hydrogen to form hydrogen gas H_2, but with another electron e^- to form the so-called "active hydrogen" H^-. The hydrogen has also filled his first electron shell with two electrons.

The active hydrogen H⁻ is very reactive, it reacts very soon with water to a hydroxide ion and hydrogen gas:

$$H^- + H_2O \rightarrow OH^- + H_2 \uparrow$$

The production of catholyte

Catholyte is strong alkaline ionised water. It is produced by adding a few grams of salt – usually common salt NaCl is used – per litre of water. It reaches a pH value up to pH 13 and a redox potential below -800 mV.

If salts are dissolved in the water, the positively charged ions are attracted by the negatively charged cathode and concentrated in the cathode chamber, the negatively charged ions migrate to the positively charged anode in the other chamber.

The dissolved positively charged ions react with the large surplus of electron – here for example dissolved sodium chloride (common salt) NaCl, where sodium ions Na^+ are concentrated in the cathode chamber.

$$2\,Na^+ + 2\,H_2O + 2\,e^- \rightarrow 2\,Na^+ + 2\,OH^- + H_2 \uparrow \rightarrow 2\,Na^+ + 2\,OH^- \rightarrow 2\,NaOH$$

and

$$Na^+ + H_2O + 2\,e^- \rightarrow Na^+ + OH^- + H + e^- \rightarrow NaOH + H^-$$

Again, the water molecule H_2O becomes a hydroxide ion OH^- and hydrogen escapes as hydrogen gas H_2 or becomes active hydrogen H^-, which again combines with water to OH^- and H_2. The OH^- ion combines with the sodium ion Na^+ to form sodium hydroxide NaOH, which in aqueous solution is caustic soda. Thus, a pH value of up to pH 13 can be achieved electrolytically.

Reactions with hard water containing lime

The above reaction differs with calcium ions Ca^{++}, which occur in drinking water, since calcium ions are twice positively charged, which means they lack two electrons:

$$Ca^{++} + 2\,H_2O + 2\,e^- \rightarrow Ca^{++} + 2\,OH^- + H_2 \uparrow \rightarrow Ca^{++} + 2\,OH^- \rightarrow Ca(OH)_2$$

and

$$Ca^{++} + 2\,H_2O + 4\,e^- \rightarrow Ca^{++} + 2\,OH^- + 2\,H + 2\,e^- \rightarrow Ca(OH)_2 + 2\,H^-$$

As in the previous reactions, the water molecule H_2O becomes the hydroxide ion OH^-, hydrogen escapes as hydrogen gas H_2 or becomes active hydrogen H^-, reacting with water to OH^- and H_2. The calcium ion Ca^{++}, however, needs two hydroxide ions OH^- for neutralization because it lacks two electrons. The calcium ion becomes calcium hydroxide $Ca(CO)_2$, as it is used as slaked lime for mortar production. Calcium salts cannot be used for the production of catholyte because they are deposited on the cathode. At higher concentrations, they quickly form an insulating layer that interrupts ionisation.

In theory, the following reactions are also possible:

$$Ca^{++} + 2\,H_2O + 3\,e^- \rightarrow Ca^{++} + 2\,OH^- + H2 \uparrow + e^- \rightarrow Ca^{++} + 2\,OH^- + e^- \rightarrow Ca(OH) + OH^-$$

and

$$Ca^{++} + 2\,H_2O + 5\,e^- \rightarrow Ca^{++} + 2\,OH^- + 2\,H + 3\,e^- \rightarrow$$
$$Ca^{++} + 2\,OH^- + 2\,H + 1\,e^- \rightarrow Ca(OH) + 2\,H^- + OH^-$$

The water molecule H_2O becomes hydroxide ion OH^-, hydrogen escapes as hydrogen gas H_2 or becomes active hydrogen H^-, reacting with water to OH^- and H_2.

The calcium ion Ca^{++} neutralizes itself with an electron e^- and with a hydroxide ion OH^-, so that one OH^- remains. Ca(OH) in combination with phosphorus as hydroxyapatite (apatite-(OH)) is the most essential component of the human skeleton.

Reactions in the anode chamber

In the anode chamber, the positively charged anode "absorbs" electrons from the water, thus resulting in a strong electron deficiency, also called positive charge or positive redox potential. This electron deficiency causes the following reactions:

$$2\,H_2O - 4\,e^- \rightarrow 4\,H^+ + O_2 \uparrow \rightarrow \downarrow 4\,H_2O \rightarrow 4\,H_3O^+$$

Through the "electron suction effect" of the positively charged anode, the two connecting electrons are detached from the water molecule H_2O and thus the connection between the two hydrogen H and the oxygen O is dissolved. The reactive oxygen O combines with a second O to form oxygen gas O_2, which dissolves in the water or degasses as bubbles.

Since the emerging H^+ ions are single protons, they cannot exist alone and always combine immediately with water H_2O to H_3O^+ molecules, making the water acidic.

If the outgassing of the oxygen is not complete, the following reactions may occur:

$$2\,H_2O - 4\,e^- \rightarrow 4\,H^+ + 2\,O \rightarrow 4\,H^+ + O_2 \rightarrow \downarrow 4\,H_2O \rightarrow 4\,H_3O^+ + O_2 \uparrow$$

and

$$3\,H_2O - 6\,e^- \rightarrow 6\,H^+ + 3\,O \rightarrow 6\,H^+ + O_3 \rightarrow \downarrow 4\,H_2O \rightarrow 6\,H_3O^+ + O_3 \uparrow$$

Dissolved elementary oxygen O, oxygen gas O_2 and ozone O_3 are produced in an acidic environment

If only one electron is removed from the H_2O molecule, an H^+ ion splits off and the very reactive and extremely strongly oxidizing hydroxyl radical HO is formed, which combines with a second HO to form a hydrogen peroxide molecule H_2O_2, a light, very strongly oxidizing acid:

$$2\,H_2O - 2\,e^- \rightarrow 2\,HO + 2\,H^+ \rightarrow H_2O_2 + 2\,H^+ \rightarrow \downarrow 4\,H_2O \rightarrow H_2O_2 + 2\,H_3O^+$$

The production of anolyte

Anolyte is strong acidic ionised water. It is also produced by adding a few grams of salt per litre of water – NaCl common salt is usually used here as well. It reaches a pH value below pH 2 and a redox potential above +1,000 mV.

If salts are dissolved in the water, the negatively charged ions are attracted by the positively charged anode and concentrated in the anode chamber, the positively charged ions migrate to the negatively charged cathode in the other chamber.

From the dissolved negatively charged ions, electrons are withdrawn. With dissolved sodium chloride (sodium chloride) NaCl, chloride ions Cl^- are concentrated in the anode chamber:

$$2\,H_2O + 2\,Cl^- - 2\,e^- \rightarrow 2\,H_2O + Cl_2 \rightarrow 2\,HOCl + 2\,H^+ \rightarrow \downarrow 2\,H_2O \rightarrow 2\,HOCl + 2\,H_3O^+$$

If electrons are removed from the chloride ions, they become elementary chlorine, which immediately reacts with water to form hypochlorous acid HOCl, a very strong oxidizing agent. In this way, a pH value below pH 2 can be achieved electrolytically.

Physical or chemical bases and acids?

There are two differences between electrolytically and chemically produced bases and acids.

Firstly, electrolytically produced bases and acids have a substantially higher or lower redox potential at the same pH value. This is shown, for example, in the following table:

Substance	pH value	redox potential
Strong alkaline water - Catholyte	pH 11.67	-245 mV
0.8% caustic soda solution	pH 11.64	+245 mV
3% ammonia solution	pH 11.62	+552 mV
Strong acidic water - Anolyte	pH 2.45	+1156 mV
0.013% hypochlorous acid	pH 2.45	+627 mV
10% acetic acid	pH 2.42	+616 mV

Table 4: Comparison of the redox potential and the pH value of electrolytically and chemically prepared bases and acids

Secondly, electrolytically produced bases and acids become "normal" water very soon, especially in the case of

- Contact with organic substances
- Dilution with normal water
- longer contact with air and light

For example, neither a catholyte with pH 12 nor an anolyte with pH 2 irritates the human skin, while both sodium hydroxide solution with pH 12 and hydrochloric acid with pH 2 cause severe damage.

Chapter 12: Alkaline mineral water ionisers

Under the term "alkaline mineral water ionisers", all water treatment devices are summarized that change the electric field of the water without an electric power supply. Alkaline mineral water ionisers, in contrast to electric water ionisers, do not need electricity, the ionisation of water is done solely by natural processes. Alkaline mineral water ionisers are available as a wide variety of products, from simple sticks inserted into a glass of water to permanently installed filter systems with complex post-processing and optimization of the water.

Mineral water ionisers offer a simple and natural way of making water alkaline and reducing, rich in hydrogen and with an antioxidant effect.

How does an alkaline mineral water ioniser work?

An alkaline mineral water ioniser contains a mineral with "loose" electrons, able to replace an H atom in one or more H_2O molecules upon contact with water. Thus, the OH^- ions formed bind to the mineral with the negatively charged oxygen side. This process releases hydrogen atoms. Best suited for this purpose is metallic magnesium Mg, which reacts with water to form Mg^{++}, releasing 2 electrons e^-, and replaces with the two released electrons in two water molecules one hydrogen atom H each by one electron e^-. The OH^- ions thus formed are then "attached" to the magnesium, forming a magnesium hydroxide molecule $Mg(OH)_2$. Two hydrogen atoms remain and combine to a gaseous hydrogen molecule H_2.

Alkaline mineral water ionisers are rooted in the tradition of East Asian medicine, where the improvement of the quality of water with combinations of minerals and metals has been known

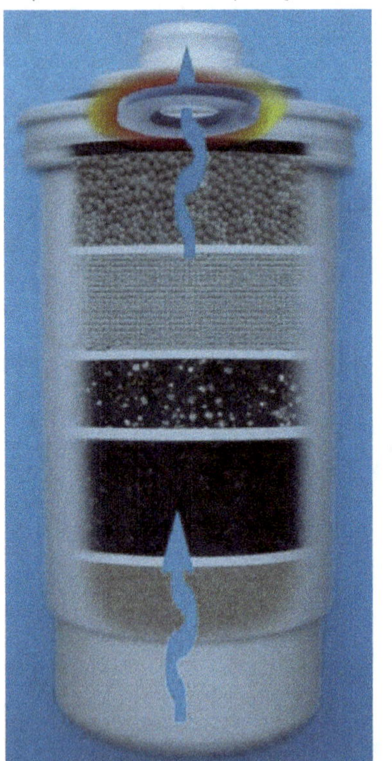

for many centuries. Recent finds date the beginning of the production of fired clay objects in China to the 15th century B.C., finds in Japan date from the 13th century B.C., from where the knowledge about the handling of clay minerals, the firing technique and the production of ceramics spreads east via Korea.

Based on this tradition, the knowledge about so-called "functional" ceramics developed, which can be used for healing purposes and also for the improvement, treatment and purification of the water. In China, for example, "red clay" has been part of traditional medicine for many centuries.

Good alkaline mineral water ionisers achieve – depending on the water quality of the input water – concentrations of hydrogen gas and negative redox potential comparable with electric water ionisers. We have measured up to pH 10 at a redox value of -400 mV.

Due to their easy handling and the comparably low price, alkaline mineral water ionisers of the new generation are certainly an option for many households.

Fig. 37: Cross section through an alkaline mineral water ioniser filter

Selection and processing of the minerals

Minerals can only react with water on their surfaces, therefore, they are usually finely ground to increase their surface and thus the contact area to the water. They are then formed to small balls about the size of peas and baked in high-temperature furnaces.

The mineral compositions are chosen depending on the desired effects of the ceramics on the water, they are different for each manufacturer and their production secret.

The components of these water ceramic balls are in various compositions:

- **Metallic magnesium** lowers the redox potential and increases the pH value of the water. This reaction is responsible for the hydrogen gas formation and the negative redox potential. *Patrick Flanagan*, the pioneer of micro-cluster research, invented the famous "Active-H", which contains nano-fine magnesium that dissolves in water and releases hydrogen.

- **Tourmaline powder**. Tourmalines are very different minerals based on silicon, they can have different colours, structures and properties depending on their trace components. They are pyroelectric and piezoelectric, which means they release electrons when their ambient temperature changes or when they are placed under voltage.

- **Zeolite powder**. Zeolites are also minerals based on silicon. They are particularly characterized by their ability to adsorb acidic substances.

- **Kaolin powder**. Kaolin is an aluminium silicate which, among other things, is the basic material for porcelain production.

- **Maifanshi powder**. Maifanshi is also an aluminium silicate with admixtures of various elements. It is of great importance in Japanese and Chinese medicine. Maifanshi can contain the most important minerals and trace elements and release them and their information structure in ionised form, depending on its composition in different proportions: Potassium, calcium, magnesium, iron, zinc, copper, molybdenum, selenium, manganese, lithium germanium, etc.

- **Magnetic iron** or magnetite. Magnets break up the cluster structures of the water, make it softer and more usable for the body.

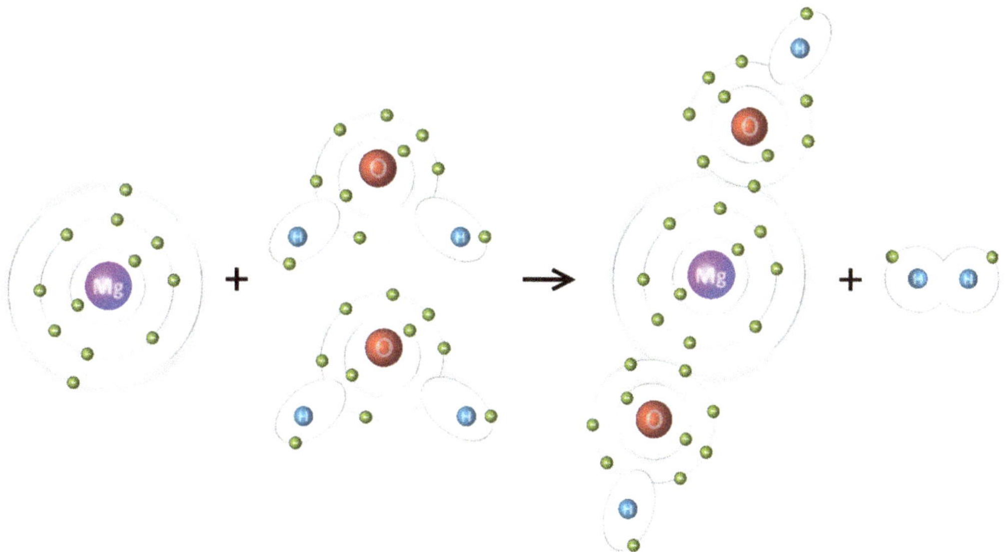

Fig. 38: Reaction in an alkaline mineral water ioniser: Mg + 2 H$_2$O → Mg(OH)$_2$ + H$_2$

Applications

Water ionisation with alkaline minerals is possible in various ways. The simplest method is to pour the water onto the alkaline mineral ceramic balls and let it interact for some time. Thus, for example, alkaline mineral ceramic balls are offered in small containers with holes, which are placed in drinking bottles, or in hollow perforated rods, with which the water can be stirred in a glass. More comfortable are filters, containing alkaline mineral ceramic balls in layers in the optimal sequence, through which the water flows, so that alkaline ionised water is available immediately and also in larger quantities.

Differences in taste

The gourmet will immediately taste the difference between an "electrically" and a "mineral" produced alkaline ionised water. Even if the same water is used and the technical measured values such as redox potential and pH value are identical, the taste of the alkaline ionised water produced the "mineral" way is often described as "round", "full" or "warm", while the alkaline ionised water produced the "electrical" way is described as "cool", "clear" or "technical", though both waters get the attributes "soft" and "palatable".

It can therefore be called a matter of taste whether electric ionised or alkaline mineral ionised water is preferred.

Chapter 13: Physical Properties

The H_2O molecule appears very simple, but has many unexpected physical properties that are important for life. One of these properties is the natural dissociation, the separation of the H_2O molecule into a negatively charged OH^- molecule and a positively charged free proton H^+, which combines to H_2OH^+ with a second water molecule. This dissociation takes place to a small extent in nature. If the dissociation rate is increased electrically and the two products are physically segregated, alkaline ionised water is produced on one side and acidic ionised water on the other.

The pH values

Alkaline ionised water from a direct flow water ioniser has a pH value (without addition of salt) between approx. pH 8 and a maximum pH 11, the simultaneously produced acidic ionised water has a pH value between approx. pH 6 and pH 3, whereby this value mainly depends on whether the local water contains acidic minerals like chlorine or sulphur.

The pH value achieved depends mainly on four factors:

- the **voltage** applied to the electrodes,
- the **conductivity** of the water,
- and the **duration** of its stay in the electrode chamber

influence the pH value: the higher the voltage, the higher the conductivity and the longer the stay of the water in the electrode chamber, the higher or lower it becomes.

The pH value can thus be increased or decreased considerably by increasing the conductivity of the water, for example by adding minerals or salts. Therefore, for the production of highly alkaline or strongly acidic "concentrate" up to pH 13 (catholyte) or pH 1 (anolyte), special direct flow ionisers are used in which a salt solution is added to the input water, or batch ionisers in which salt can be dissolved.

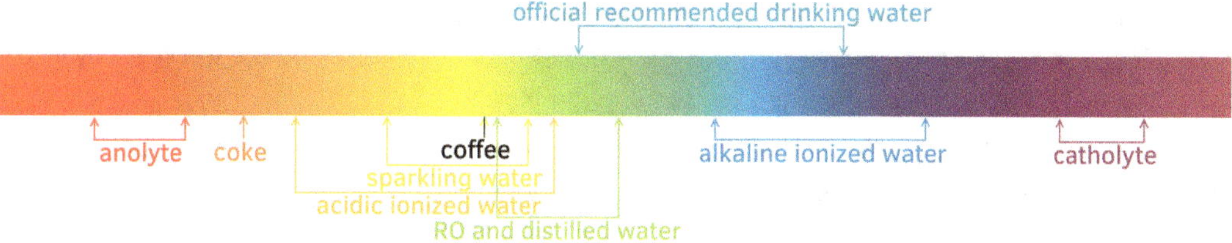

Fig 39: Typical pH values in different liquids

The redox potential

Alkaline ionised water has a strongly negative, acidic ionised water a strongly positive redox potential. How high or low the redox potential of the ionised water becomes, also depends on many factors, including the conductivity of the water and the strength of the voltage applied to the electrodes, but also the shape of the electrodes and other factors. A decrease of the redox potential is always associated with the "production" of hydrogen and oxygen gas by decomposing water molecules.

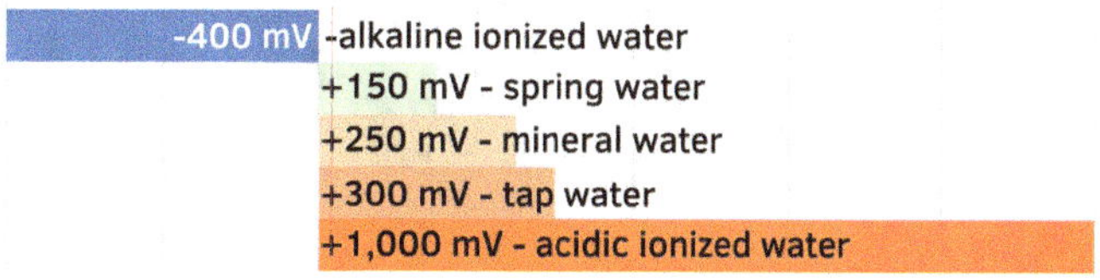

Fig. 40: Typical redox values in different waters

-400 mV - alkaline ionized water
+150 mV - spring water
+250 mV - mineral water
+300 mV - tap water
+1,000 mV - acidic ionized water

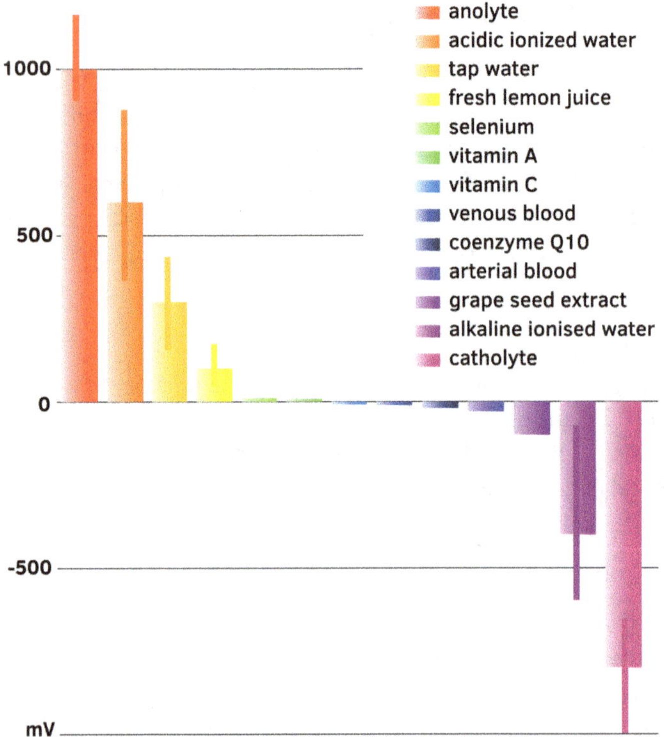

Fig. 41: Redox values of different substances

Small water clusters

The size of water clusters depends on the number of water molecules per water cluster and therefore varies greatly. In tap water, clusters contain many hundreds of molecules, in spring and stream water they are very small, as well as in ionised water from a water ioniser.

The number of water clusters can be determined and calculated by NMR analysis (Nuclear Magnetic Resonance Spectroscopy) by measuring the resonance frequencies. Ionised water has a resonance frequency at 53 Hz, the same as a living human cell.

Hexagonal water molecules are – as Korean research shows – one of the fundamentals for a healthy cell environment. This research shows that hexagonal water has much higher solubility, energy and transport capacities than "normal" water and that the percentage of hexagonal water in the human body decreases with its perceived and biological ageing. In regions where people age healthily and slowly, hexagonal water often found. In nature, hexagonal water comes from artesian wells, springs or glaciers. Technically, it can be produced by certain forms of vortex or ionisation. Ionised water from a water ioniser is water with a very high proportion of hexagonal water structure.

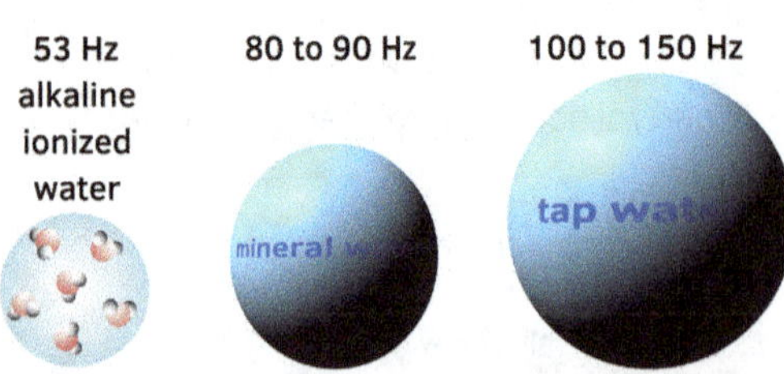

Fig. 42: Water cluster size measurement by NMR

Dietmar Ferger • Fountain of Youth Water

Electrical Ionisation - A Summary

Only in conductive water, ionisation is possible, therefore, dissolved salts must be in the water, which are present in ionic form, for example like Na^+ and Cl^-.

At the **negatively charged electrode** of an electric water ioniser, **electrons are released into the water**. These electrons attach themselves to the positively charged alkaline mineral ions like calcium Ca^{++} and magnesium Mg^+, so that these are neutralized or negatively charged. At the same time, the negatively charged acidic mineral ions such as chlorine Cl^-, nitrate NO_3^- and sulphur S^- are attracted by the positive charge of the other electrode and migrate through the selective membrane into the other half of the ionisation unit.

At the same time, the electrons "banish" one H atom out of water molecules, one electron replaces one H at the H_2O molecule, OH^- ions and hydrogen atoms H are formed. A hydrogen atom can now either unite with a second hydrogen to form a hydrogen molecule H_2 (hydrogen gas), or it receives a second electron from the electron pool and becomes a so-called "active hydrogen" H^-. A part of the hydrogen gas becomes microbubbles and pearls out of the glass, the rest dissolves in the water by placing the tiny hydrogen gas molecules between the water molecules.

A high electron density can result from the coupling to hydrogen, since hydrogen is the smallest atom and so many electrons can be contained in the smallest space. If a hydrogen atom with 1 g/mole or a hydrogen gas molecule with 2 g/mole transports an additional electron, this is about 180 or 90 times as much per gram as vitamin C with 176 g/mole.

This, a strong negative charge can be measured in alkaline ionised water, but its electrons cannot be assigned exactly. Alkaline ionised water is therefore a strong reducing agent.

At the **positively charged electrode** of an electric water ioniser, **electrons are removed from the water**. This oxidizes the negatively charged acidic minerals such as chlorine Cl^-, nitrate NO_3^- or sulphur S^- so that they are neutralized or positively charged. The positively charged alkaline minerals like calcium Ca^{++} and magnesium Mg^+ are attracted by the other electrode and migrate through the membrane into the other half of the ionisation unit.

At the same time, from H_2O molecules binding electrons are removed, creating H^+ ions (protons) and oxygen atoms. Two or three oxygen atoms combine to form oxygen gas O_2 or ozone O_3, which dissolves in the water or gasses out. The protons combine with water molecules to form H_2OH^+, also written as H^+. Oxygen and ozone molecules as well as a lack of electrons cause a strong oxidation capability, which is increased by the hypochlorous acid HOCl, which develops in the presence of chloride. Thus, a strong positive charge can be measured in acidic ionised water; it is a strong oxidizing agent.

Chapter 14: Biological properties of alkaline ionised water

Due to its special physical characteristics, alkaline ionised water also has special effects. Used as daily drinking water, it gradually changes the structure of the body water – the lymph and the connective tissue fluid – and thus the structure and overall condition of the body. The body's own processes and mechanisms are changed or made possible again.

This lays the foundation for an efficient transport of substances in the body and a sufficient supply of free electrons.

Chemical and physical bases or acids

It is important for understanding the biological effect that alkaline and acidic ionised water are **physically produced solutions**. This means that the pH value is achieved physically and not chemically by adding chemicals or minerals. The OH^- or H^+ ions are therefore "free" or "unbuffered", they have no "corresponding" chemical in the water.

For further explanation: if alkaline water is produced chemically, for example by adding sodium carbonate Na_2CO_3, then the following reaction occurs:

$$Na_2CO_3 + H_2O \rightarrow 2Na^+ + HCO_3 + OH^- \leftrightarrow NaHCO_3 + NaOH.$$

In this reaction, the strong base sodium hydroxide NaOH and the weak base sodium hydrogen carbonate $NaHCO_3$ are formed, but there are no "free" OH^- ions and also no free hydrogen as they are formed during the electrolytic separation of H_2O into OH^- and hydrogen gas H_2.

In our body, this makes a decisive difference in the physiological effect: While NaOH or any other "chemical" base neutralizes the gastric acid HCl by forming a salt NaCl:

$$NaOH + HCl \leftrightarrow Na^+ + Cl^- + H_2O \leftrightarrow NaCl + H_2O$$

with alkaline ionised water containing only a free OH^- ion, the stomach acid remains untouched, since chlorine cannot form salt with an OH^- ion:

$$OH^- + HCl \leftrightarrow OH^- + H^+ + Cl^- \leftrightarrow Cl^- + H_2O.$$

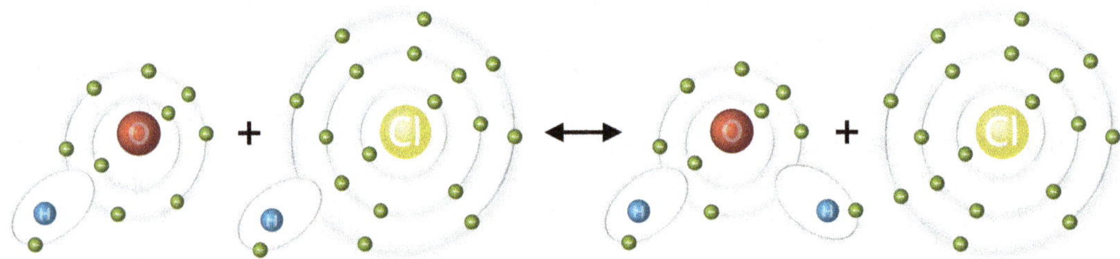

Fig. 43: alkaline ionised water does not neutralize gastric or hydrochloric acid

Alkaline ionised water regulates gastric acid

In Japan and Korea, drinking alkaline ionised water is generally recommended for all kinds of **digestive problems**. *(See also Chapter 9: Development in Japan and Korea, page 49)*

If drinking alkaline ionised water, it gets into the stomach first. There, it regulates gastric acid HCl by slightly reducing an excess of H^+ ions, but not neutralizing the gastric acid itself. In people with too much gastric acid, the excess acid is reduced (but without chemically neutralising it), in people with too little gastric acid, the cells in the stomach are stimulated to produce more HCl, thus increasing the acid level.

Alkaline ionised water relieves the pancreas

Drink alkaline ionised water on an empty stomach!

Especially in the morning, the parietal cells – the cells in the stomach producing the gastric acid – are still "asleep". They are not activated by water as long as it does not contain additives such as carbonic acid, sugar or flavourings. Thus, pure water can reach the pylorus at the lower end of the stomach without contact to gastric acid, which otherwise would "swallow" most OH^- ions.

Provided the stomach musculature is intact, an empty stomach is a tube about 20 cm / 8 inch long, only expanding when "digestible" contents enter. The pylorus is the sphincter muscle of the stomach, separating the stomach from the intestine. It detects that pure water does not need digestion and opens up, allowing the alkaline ionised water to reach the small intestine undiluted.

Thus, the small intestine becomes hydrated, the **pancreas is relieved**.

The task of the pancreas is to neutralise the acidic chyme by injecting alkaline secretion – it is the counterpart of the parietal cells. It produces sodium hydroxide NaOH from the sodium bicarbonate $NaHCO_3$ in the blood and water H_2O, leaving carbonic acid H_2CO_3 remaining in the blood.

This reaction lowers the pH value of the blood, which, for example, is the main reason why we get tired after eating.

Drinking alkaline ionised water – especially in the morning on an empty stomach – makes the small intestine more alkaline, energized and hydrated, the pancreas needs less sodium bicarbonate and less carbon dioxide is produced in the blood. This also reduces or eliminates the typical **performance slump** after a meal.

Alkaline ionised water is an antioxidant.

Due to its strongly negative redox potential, alkaline ionised water is a **strong reducing agent** or antioxidant. Japanese researchers prove that alkaline ionised water with a redox potential of -100 to -700 mV is able to neutralize the free radicals in the body with its excess electrons and its content of hydrogen gas.

Alkaline ionised water is energy water

Electrons are a physical form of energy.

If we drink mineral or tap water with a lack of electrons, our body has to supply electrons to the water before it can absorb it. If the body suffers from a lack of energy or electrons and cannot energize the water, it cannot absorb the water properly, it may enter the connective tissues, but cannot hydrate the cells.

Therefore, we can drink a lot of "normal" water, but our body cannot use it properly because water absorption means losing energy. Perhaps it is one reason for the disappearance of thirst in seniors, that their body intelligence is "frustrated" by years of drinking non-usable water and has learned that drinking water costs a lot of energy, which has to be used sparingly – especially in old age.

The increase in energy achieved by drinking electron-rich alkaline ionised water can be very well demonstrated by imaging techniques such as Kirlian photography. Also, all analysis devices measuring the conductivity of the body meridians based on skin resistance measurements at the acupuncture points – like electroacupuncture according to Voll – often show positive reactions and improvements within a few minutes after drinking alkaline ionised water.

Alkaline ionised water and antioxidant diet

The increased intake of antioxidants is controversial nowadays. It has been shown that artificial antioxidants like ascorbic acid interfere with the immune system and tend to have negative long-term effects, especially because they themselves become oxidizing agents after they release their electrons. However, vitamin-rich food is an indispensable source of health. Unfortunately, caused by bad and acidic environmental influences, the vitamin content in vegetables and fruit decreases more and more and industrial processing lowers it even further.

The strength of an antioxidant and its reducing effect depends on the molecular weight of the antioxidant or reducing agent: the lower the molecular weight, the stronger it is. If water molecules with molecular weight 18 carry electrons, the electron density is considerably higher than if vitamin C molecules with molecular weight 176 carries an electron each. Furthermore, one can drink water nearly without limit, but food and antioxidant intake are very limited.

Substance	Molecular weight
Alkaline ionised water molecule	18
Beta-carotene	150
Vitamin E	153
Vitamin C	176

Table 5: comparison of molecular weight

Alkaline ionised water promotes a healthy intestinal microflora

A healthy microflora of the small intestine is an essential prerequisite for a functioning nutrient absorption, an intact immune system and overall good health.

In the upper part of the small intestine, the intestinal microflora consists mainly of various basophilic bacterial strains, which symbiotically break down and utilize the ingested food. They are mainly destroyed by antibiotics, nevertheless, a permanently too acidic environment can also weaken them and promote the colonisation of acidophilic fungi. An acidic milieu is mainly caused by a "normal" diet with high acid surplus, which leads to a lack of sodium bicarbonate in the blood. This deficiency **overstrains the pancreas**, which cannot completely neutralise the acidic food chyme coming from the stomach, so that the intestinal environment shifts into the acidic range. Therefore, drinking alkaline ionised water also contributes to stable intestinal health and thus to a stable immune system.

Alkaline ionised water promotes blood circulation

In healthy state, the erythrocytes, the red blood cells, are electrically negatively charged, thus, they repel each other and do not clump together. In an oxidized organism, the erythrocytes lack the electrons, they lose their charge. In a neutral state they no longer repel each other and clump together, therefore, the blood becomes thicker.

Microwave radiation from mobile phones, Wi-Fi and so on are one of the main causes of clumped erythrocytes.

By drinking alkaline ionised water, erythrocytes regain their electrical charge in a relatively short time – in some cases within a few hours –, the clumping is eliminated and blood circulation improved. Even high blood pressure can be lowered by the "dilution" of the blood and the reduction of arterial "calcification" caused by plaques.

Alkaline ionised water improves connective tissue

Over-acidified connective tissues are the cause of many skin and subcutaneous problems. Drinking alkaline ionised water slowly increases the pH value of the connective tissues – you can follow this process by measuring the saliva pH value. By increasing the pH of the connective tissues, their capillaries are opened up, thus improving the supply with oxygen and nutrients.

Due to better blood circulation in the connective tissues, the skin cells are also better supplied and moisturized from the inside. This has direct effects on the appearance of skin: the skin does not dry out so fast, remains more elastic and forms fewer wrinkles. This also reduces the susceptibility to sunburn. Furthermore, the tightening and better blood circulation of the connective tissues also reduces **cellulite** or stops it from developing. Cellulite is a deformation of the deeper layers of the subcutaneous and connective tissues that is usually resistant to therapy, it cannot really be eliminated or smoothed by any treatment, cream, massage or liposuction.

Alkaline ionised water stops tooth decay

Despite improved dental hygiene, electric toothbrushes and fluoridated toothpastes, caries diseases are becoming increasingly common. Caries is caused by bacteria like Streptococcus mutans, breaking down sugar and simple carbohydrates into acids. Since these bacteria prefer an acidic environment, they feel very comfortable in acidic saliva. If the saliva becomes more alkaline – which is usually the case with regular drinking of alkaline ionised water and limited sugar and white flour consumption – the environment becomes "uncomfortable" for the caries-forming bacteria, so that they can no longer develop well and their metabolic activity and thus the production of acids is reduced.

Alkaline ionised water prevents rusting

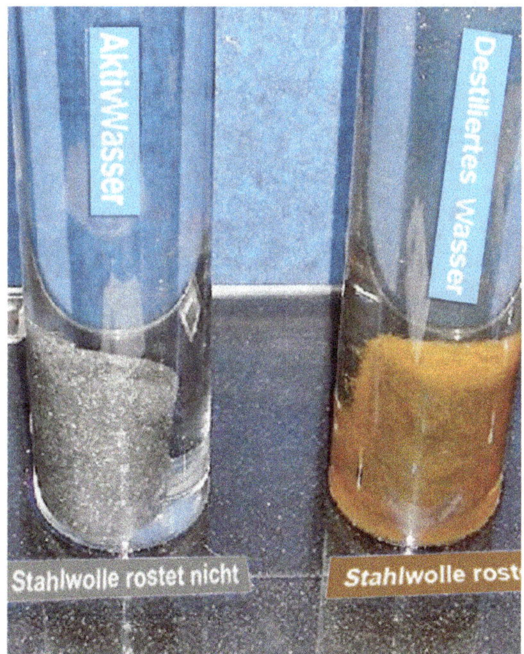

Alkaline ionised water can be used as an effective rust inhibitor:

Steel wool rusts in normal water, but not in alkaline active water. Rusting is a slow form of oxidation; an explosion would be the fastest. There are many levels in between, because oxidation can affect many materials and substances – we know the following processes:

- Iron rusts.
- Proteins become denatured.
- Oils and fats become rancid.
- Apples turn brown.
- Carbohydrates burn

These are all oxidation processes.

Fig. 44: Steel wool does not rust in alkaline ionised water

Alkaline ionised water is oxygen-rich water.

In alkaline ionised water, the concentration of OH⁻ ions is ten times higher at pH 8 and ten thousand times higher at pH 11 than in neutral water. Each of these OH⁻ ions lacks a hydrogen atom, which leads to an **excess of oxygen**. The oxygen stored in alkaline ionised water serves the body as an **oxygen depot** available at any time and can be recalled as oxygen gas O_2 by the self-reaction shown below. In a reaction of 4 OH⁻ ions to two H_2O molecules not only one molecule of the oxygen gas O_2 is formed, but also 4 electrons, it is an energy-producing reaction that can buffer free radicals in the body.

As soon as the lymph has an alkaline pH value, it becomes an oxygen depot from which oxygen can be retrieved at any time, for example for sporting activities, without oxidative stress.

The fact that alkaline water and lymph is a non-oxidizing oxygen depot has already saved our lives. A growing foetus in the mother's womb swims in alkaline amniotic fluid, so that a child has a thoroughly alkaline body at birth – for good reason:

Since cutting the umbilical cord abruptly stops the oxygen supply from the mother's blood, but the lungs have not yet reached their full functional capacity and have to unfold slowly, a child would suffocate immediately after birth if it were unable to extract oxygen from its alkaline body fluid.

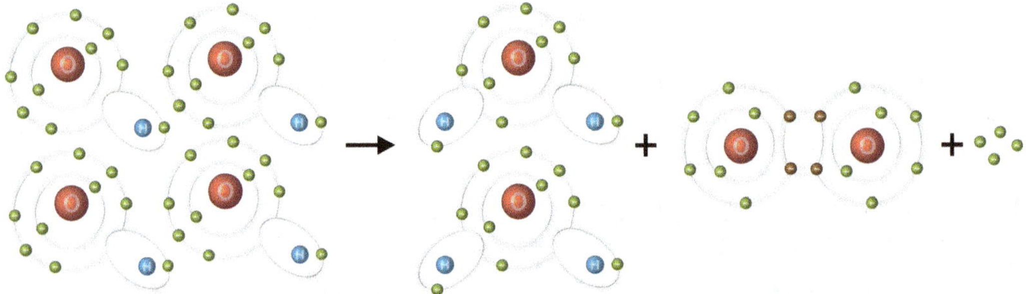

Fig. 45: Alkaline ionised water provides oxygen and electrons

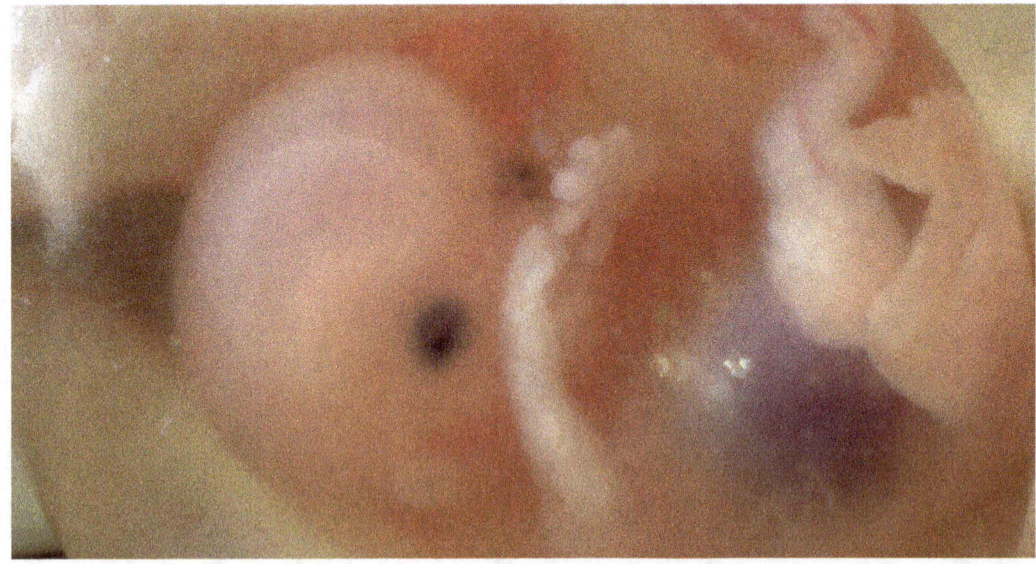

Fig. 46: The growing foetus swims in alkaline water
(Source: Wikimedia commons, drsuparna, Jacopo Werther)

Chapter 15: Biological properties of acidic ionised water

Acidic ionised water is a by-product of electric water ionisers. The Russian researchers called it "water of death", since it is hostile to life and kills certain organisms – especially micro-organisms. Acidic ionised water, which is produced in industrial ionisers with the addition of salt, has strong disinfecting and antibiotic properties. It is then called "anolyte" because it is formed at the anode of the electrolysis chamber.

Anolyte is an oxidizing and disinfecting agent

Due to their excess of H^+ ions, acidic ionised water and anolyte are oxidizing agents, they rob other molecules of electrons and thus of energy. This energy drain weakens unicellular organisms and ultimately kills them. Therefore, anolyte is effective against many micro-organisms attacking the human immune system.

Anolyte, which is acidic ionised water produced with the addition of common salt NaCl, has four mechanisms for killing microorganisms:

- Anolyte has a redox potential of more than +1,000 mV to attack the cell membranes of microorganisms, oxidizing them and finally make them die.
- With a pH value below pH 3, anolyte destroys the cell walls weakened by oxidation.
- Proteins are denatured with active chlorine.
- Anolyte contains hydroxyl radicals HO· and hydrogen peroxide H_2O_2, by-products of its production. These are also strong oxidizing agents, attacking the cell walls.

Anolyte does not chemically attack microorganisms, but strip them of electrons. Hence the formation of resistance to anolyte – in contrast to chemical antibiotics – is virtually impossible.

Anolyte can therefore be used effectively to combat the following microorganisms, among others, without developing resistance and without side effects:

- **Staphylococcus aureus**, bacteria causing pneumonia and skin infections. They are latently present in about 25% of the population.
- **Staphylococcus epidermis**, bacteria often occurring in hospitals and exhibiting a resistance rate to standard antibiotics of 70%. They can cause life-threatening inflammation in people with a weakened immune system after surgery.
- **Pseudomonas aeruginosa**, also a widespread hospital germ resistant to many antibiotics. It is also causing severe inflammation.
- **Streptococcus mutans**, bacteria in the oral cavity causing tooth decay by feeding on glucose and excreting lactic acid that softens the enamel and thus paves the way for caries bacteria.
- **Escherichia coli**, bacteria that are vital and useful in the intestines, but which can lead to serious diseases in other parts of the body, for example in the urinary tract.
- **Enterococci**, bacteria useful in the intestine, but which are also found in infectious surgical wounds and inflammations of the diabetic foot.
- **Salmonella enteritidis**, bacteria that cause severe intestinal diseases in humans and trigger diarrhoea and nausea.

- **Salmonella typhi**, bacteria which cause typhoid fever, a feverish disease with severe diarrhoea.

- **Shigella flexneri**, bacteria which cause the so-called bacterial dysentery, which is often characterized by bloody diarrhoea and severe abdominal pain.

- **Trichophyton rubrum**, resistant filamentous fungi which can cause severe skin diseases.

- **Candida albicans**, fungi which cause the so-called candidiasis or thrush, which appears on the mucous membranes, on the genitals, in the intestines or on the skin. Candida albicans fungi are present in about 3/4 of all humans, but are kept in check by a functioning immune system.

- **Herpes simplex**, viruses which cause the herpes diseases.

- **Polioviruses**, the pathogens causing poliomyelitis or polio.

- **Coxsackie viruses**, which cause flu-like symptoms and can lead to meningitis and heart muscle inflammation.

The following study was conducted at Kitatsato University in Tokyo, one of Japan's best-known universities: Using anolyte with a pH of 2.5, a redox potential of 1125 mV and a chlorine content of 40 ppm, various microorganisms were treated for the specified period of time, then they were neutralized and the remaining colonies were counted. It shows that with the exception of the multi-resistant and omnipresent, but mostly harmless Bacillus subtilis, all germs – including multi-resistant hospital germs – are killed by anolyte in a maximum exposure time of 30 seconds:

Bacteria time	start	5 sec	30 sec	60 sec	10 min	30 min	60 min
Staphylococcus aureus	$4,5 \times 10^5$	2	0	0	0	0	0
Methizillin-resistent Staphyllococcus aureus	$1,4 \times 10^5$	10	0	0	0	0	0
Escherichia coli	$4,2 \times 10^5$	0	0	0	0	0	0
Pseudomonas aeruginosa	$8,2 \times 10^5$	0	0	0	0	0	0
Bacillus subtilis	$1,0 \times 10^5$	1000	1000	1000	1000	4	0
Fungi							
Trichophyton rubrum	$2,0 \times 10^3$	1	0	0	0	0	0
Candida albicans	$2,4 \times 10^3$	0	0	0	0	0	0
Viruses							
Herpes	$4,0 \times 10^4$	0	0	0	0	0	0
Polio	$4,6 \times 10^4$	0	0	0	0	0	0
Coxsackie	$4,3 \times 10^4$	0	0	0	0	0	0

Table 6: Effect of anolyte with 40 ppm chlorine content on various microorganisms

For comparison, the effect of the most common disinfectant sodium hypochlorite NaClO, also with a chlorine content of 40 ppm, was tested on some of the listed microorganisms. NaClO is used, for example, to disinfect swimming pools and in dentistry for root canal treatment. The results were as follows:

   Dietmar Ferger • Fountain of Youth Water

Bacteria time	start	5 sec	30 sec	60 sec
Staphylococcus aureus	$4{,}5 \times 10^5$	2600	630	290
Methizillin-resistent Staphyllococcus aureus	$1{,}4 \times 10^5$	1900	250	10
Escherichia coli	$4{,}2 \times 10^5$	2000	8,5	0
Fungi				
Candida albicans	$2{,}4 \times 10^3$	1700	0	0
Virus				
Polio	$4{,}6 \times 10^4$	5,5	0	0

Table 7: For comparison, the effect of sodium hypochlorite with 40 ppm chlorine content on selected microorganisms

Anolyte in medical practice

Due to its disinfectant, bactericidal and fungicidal properties, anolyte can be used as an effective and side-effect-free alternative to chemical disinfectants. It works by direct contact with bacteria and fungi and is particularly useful in the external treatment of:

- neurodermatitis, also in children
- psoriasis
- itchy skin
- Acne and other skin impurities
- fungal diseases of the skin
- dermatoses
- tonsillitis
- poorly healing and open wounds
- skin injuries
- diabetic feet
- Pressure points, e.g. due to lying for too long
- Sensitive gums and gum diseases

In general anolyte is used externally, for example for rinsing, washing, gargling, bathing or for compresses, and only as long as the infestation with microorganisms or inflammation is present. External treatment with anolyte should always be accompanied by internal detoxification and drinking of alkaline ionised water. In the case of severe diarrhoea, acidic ionised water or diluted anolyte can also be drunk for the duration of the illness. For this, at least one large glass should be drunk in one go on an empty stomach so that the water reaches the intestines and does not "get stuck" in the stomach.

Anolyte is also very well suited for disinfecting large areas, as its use in China, for example, in the fight against coronavirus shows – in "western" societies, influenced by the pharmaceutical industry, expensive chemical disinfectants that are harmful to the environment and to the water are used instead.

Anolyte in animal and plant breeding

Anolyte is also used very successfully in innovative livestock farming operations. The fields of application are manifold:

Adding 3 to 8 % of anolyte to the drinking water of fattening animals – such as pigs – improves feed conversion, health and meat quality, antibiotics rarely or never need to be used.

Nebulizing a low-percentage anolyte solution in the barn reduces the germ pressure significantly, the air becomes better and bad odours disappear.

Chapter 16: Answers to frequently asked questions

In the many years that I have been working with ionised water, I have been asked hundreds of questions about the effects and properties of alkaline and acidic ionised water.
I hope that you will also find answers to your questions here.

Who can and should drink alkaline ionised water?

Basically, anybody can drink alkaline ionised water. In the case of organic diseases like heart diseases, kidney dysfunctions etc. you should consult your doctor or practitioner before drinking alkaline ionised water.

Babies and small children can be nourished very well with weak alkaline ionised water, it is also very suitable for the production of baby food.

Older children can drink alkaline ionised water without any problems, albeit with a slightly lower pH value than adults. In our experience, children enjoy drinking this water very much and lose the desire for acidic drinks such as sparkling water or soft drinks.

Alkaline ionised water is particularly suitable for **pregnant women**. During pregnancy the expectant mother needs a lot of energy and alkaline substances, because the growing child grows up in an alkaline amniotic fluid and withdraws the required alkaline substances from the body of the expectant mother.

The mother's body gives the foetus a clear priority over its own supply and therefore provides it with all necessary alkaline substances. A healthy amniotic fluid has an alkaline pH and a pleasant smell, but midwives report that in more and more cases it stinks and is acidic - especially among smoking women - and that babies who come from acidic amniotic fluid often show skin problems and allergic reactions.

Alkaline deficiency, for example, is the cause of a pregnant woman's malaise, which usually occurs in the morning.

There are reports from Japan confirming very good experiences with alkaline ionised water for pregnant women. It is ideal for the health of the growing foetus if women start drinking alkaline ionised water at least 6 months before pregnancy, combined with other detoxification measures.

It is not recommended to start drinking alkaline ionised water during pregnancy, as its detoxifying effect may lead to acid floods in the body which could harm the foetus.

Alkaline ionised water can also be helpful for **senior citizens**, as they often suffer from dehydration and drink far too little water. This can be caused by the body's lack of energy, which no longer has enough electrons to "charge" normal electron-deficient water. Since alkaline ionised water supplies the body with free electrons, seniors often like to drink more water again.

Athletes can benefit from drinking alkaline ionised water because it increases the amount of oxygen available in the body and thus improves the supply of oxygen to the muscles without increasing the oxidation potential and the risk of ROS (reactive oxygen species). Hobby athletes are also reported to have less muscle soreness and to recover more quickly.

As Japanese studies and reports from hospitals show, drinking alkaline ionised water also supports the **healing and recovery process** for almost all diseases.

What should I bear in mind when drinking alkaline ionised water?

The most important "drink" of the day is **in the morning immediately after getting up**: Drink at least ½ litres of fresh, if necessary slightly warm alkaline ionised water - preferably before the aroma of coffee or breakfast bacon stimulates your saliva production. If you haven't eaten a thick steak the evening before, in the morning your stomach is empty and a thin tube, its parietal cells are still "sleeping" and the water gets directly into the small intestine, hydrating and alkalizing it and thus supporting the pancreas.

In order to **warm** alkaline ionised water, fill a glass with a large amount of alkaline ionised water fresh from the water ioniser and add a small amount of hot water. If you heat it directly, the majority of the free electrons and hydrogen will be "boiled out".

Different from dissolved alkaline mineral powders, alkaline ionised water does not neutralize gastric acid, therefore, you can drink it before or during meals.

It is recommended to drink 30 ml of (alkaline ionised) water per kg body weight daily, (which equals to about 2.5 ounce of water per pound body weight) plus up to 100% more for heat, heating air, salty food or heavy physical work or sports. There is no limit for drinking alkaline ionised water.

An easy method to determine whether enough water has been drunk is to observe the **colour of the urine**. This should be as colourless as possible at least once a day. The more yellow the urine, the higher the concentration of uric acid. The observation of the colour of the urine also shows if toxins and other deposits in the body are dissolved and excreted by detoxification measures. It makes sense to increase the drinking amount until the urine becomes clear again.

According to Japanese recommendations and Russian studies, the optimal pH value of alkaline ionised water for drinking is **between pH 9 to 9.5**. It is not important to maintain an exact pH value, an accuracy of $\pm$ 0.5 pH is sufficient - daily measurement is therefore not necessary. However, do not rely on displays on your water ioniser, these can be very inaccurate, since the pH and redox values displayed are not measured, but only calculated.

Drink alkaline ionised water **as fresh as possible**, as hydrogen and free electrons are very volatile. Under laboratory conditions, the redox potential had risen from an initial value of -400 mV to -200 mV after 8 hours, the outgassing of hydrogen from the water occurs much faster. The high pH value lasts somewhat longer and is lowered primarily by the carbon dioxide content of the air, but also decreases over time in closed vessels. All these values are strongly dependent on environmental influences as heat, agitation, electromagnetic fields, light etc. can strongly accelerate processes.

It should be noted that at the beginning some **violent body reactions** can occur (but do not have to). Headaches or migraines, diarrhoea and joint pain can occur because the detoxification reactions of the body are too intense. In this case, it is advisable to drink no less, but weaker alkaline ionised water with around pH 8 and gradually increase its strength. Supporting measures can also alleviate initial reactions.

If the alkaline ionised water is slightly cloudy when it is "tapped" and fine bubbles form that rise upwards, then this is excess hydrogen, which slowly outgas as hydrogen gas H_2 - drink it together with the water. If you leave the full glass to stand for a while, bubbles will form again and settle on the glass wall. However, this is oxygen gas O_2, which is released by the decreasing ionisation, the discharge and disappearance of the free electrons.

How can I determine the effect of alkaline ionised water?

If you want to observe the effect of alkaline active water, pay attention to the following parameters:

- Observe your **thirst** or desire for water. Depending on which drinks and (mineral) waters you have drunk so far, do test them whether you still like them or not.
- Observe the **colour and smell of your urine**.
- Observe the **regularity of the bowel movement** and the colour and smell of the stool.
- Observe your **need to sleep**. Sleep is mainly used for deacidification and recharging the body. If you deacidify and recharge your body with alkaline ionised water, you need less sleep.
- Smell the **air in your bedroom** in the morning. Overnight we excrete acids as gas.
- Observe your **fitness**, for example the ability to climb stairs without a break or to walk longer distances.
- Observe the appearance of **muscle soreness** during sports and how quickly it disappears.
- Observe your **skin**, especially in "problem zones".
- Observe your **connective tissue**, especially in problem areas such as thighs or upper arms.
- Observe your **appetite for sweets**.
- Observe the new **formation of tartar** during your annual visit to the dentist.

If you want to have objective measurements or visible images, the following measurements and values are very helpful:

- The **pH value of your saliva**. To measure it, wait 3 hours after the last meal, swallow the saliva three times and spit the newly formed saliva onto a pH measuring strip.
- The **blood pressure** (blood pressure measurement)
- **Heart rate** under stress (exercise ECG)
- **Heart Rate Variability** (HRV)
- The **oxygen partial pressure** pO2 of your blood (pO2 measurement in the blood)
- The **redox value of your blood** (redox value determination in the blood).
- The **lung volume** (lung function test).
- The **clotting of blood cells** (dark field microscopic image).
- The **energy field** of the body (Kirlian photography)
- The **energy potential** of the body (energy measurement by different energetic measuring methods, e.g. according to Voll)

How do I support the effect of alkaline ionised water?

Alkaline ionised water promotes general well-being and has a positive effect on almost all known health-promoting measures. Therefore, the question should be:

Which health-promoting measures can be supported by drinking alkaline ionised water - and the answer is simple.

Since it is recommended to drink a lot of water with all health-promoting measures and all long-term health programs also promote detoxification, drinking alkaline ionised water supplements all health-promoting measures and health programs.

Dr Irlacher, spa and bath doctor in Bad Fuessing in Bavaria, Germany, and other therapists in Germany, Europe, Asia and the USA impressively describe this in various publications and articles.

To support detoxification and self-cleaning of the body by drinking alkaline ionised water, we recommend:

- **Self-improvement** for stress tolerance. Since stress and psychological imbalance are very strong acidifying agents, a deliberate training of mental tolerance and balance, supported by meditation, yoga, Tai-Chi etc., can also have a very positive and acid-reducing effect.

- **Recreational sport**: we recommend regular jumping on a soft trampoline. All sports that stimulate the flow of lymph in the body promote detoxification and purification.

- **Alkaline baths**: The skin, the largest excretory organ, excretes toxins and excess acids in an alkaline bath.

- **Alkaline body care**: the skin's ability to excrete is strengthened by consistent alkaline body care. It should be noted that alkaline cosmetics are easily perishable as they do not contain any bacteria-inhibiting acids. Nevertheless, it should be free of preservatives. In the case of bacterial inflammations (e.g. acne) or allergies, acid skin care and acid ionised water or anolyte can exceptionally be used as a therapeutic agent.

- **Pulsating magnetic field resonance therapy**: It can strengthen, rearrange and harmonize the positive body signals and harmonizes particularly well with alkaline ionised water. It works by the body resonating on the impulses sent, which is all the better, the more electrons and ions are present.

- **Sauna visits**, especially in an infrared cabin, accelerates the excretion through the skin, expands the capillaries and brings the lymph into flow.

- **Hydro resonance or detox foot baths**: to be performed only by specialists. They are a highly effective method of removing toxins from the body via the foot meridians. However, as they influence the entire "body electric", this therapy should only be carried out under the supervision an experienced therapist.

- **Vitality patches**: Toxins are excreted via the body meridians ending in the soles of the foot. At the same time the whole body is activated by effective substances in the vitality patches.

- **Bloodletting**: for example, through blood donations. The increased formation of new blood improves the quality of the blood and its ability to be transported.

- **Oral hygiene**: Mouth and tongue cleansing through tongue scraping and oil pulling. The oral cavity is the place with the most bacteria in the human body.

- **Colon hydrotherapy**: professional intestinal cleansing. Deposits can form in the intestine, which promote rot and fermentation processes. Professional bowel cleansing can loosen many blockages and set processes in motion.

- **Comprehensive mineral supply**: Food supplements. After over a century of acid rain and "conventional" soil fertilization, there are hardly any trace elements left in our soils. Thus, even organically cultivated plants can no longer contain them. In the millions of years of evolution, however, our body has adapted to the substances of the periodic table and needs them, even if it is only for catalytic functions. Hence a comprehensive mineral supply through plant-bound mineral trace elements is indispensable, which should contain as many as possible of the 70 substances of the periodic table of elements.

- **Detoxification agents** for the intestines like modified lava stone (zeolite, clinoptilolite). They can bind toxins in the intestine and thus prevent the formation of harmful gases and the resulting poisoning without being absorbed by the body.
- **Alkaline green food supplement**: made from algae, alfalfa, vegetables and green cereal grasses, which contain many alkaline and detoxifying substances.
- **Blood group diet**: The blood groups differ by different sugars on the blood cells. They cause a different absorption capacity and compatibility of the different nutrients. Nutrition that is not adapted to the blood group can trigger intolerances and symptoms of auto-intoxication.
- **Glyconutrients**: The 8 essential sugars should be supplied by the diet; however, they are often – also because of the decrease of the food quality – not sufficiently present. A lack of glyconutrients causes malfunctions of the body and - as with a diet that is not adapted to the blood group - intolerances and symptoms of self-poisoning.

In addition, sufficient exercise, enough sleep and a biological diet that is as low in harmful substances as possible are of course the foundation of a healthy lifestyle.

Do I lose weight with alkaline ionised water?

Alkaline ionised water can help you lose weight. However, many deposits in connective and fatty tissue are difficult to dissolve in water. Therefore, further supporting measures are recommended for losing weight.

Prof Vincent and Dr Walker recommend low-mineral water

Louis-Claude Vincent (1906 - 1988), professor for geology and hydrology, researched the correlation between health and water quality in France in the middle of the 20th century. He found, that soft water with a low redox potential, as it occurs in the hills of the French low mountain ranges, can be connected with low mortality, whereas hard water with a high redox potential, as it is common in the industrialised plains and river valleys of France, is accompanied by high mortality. It is a characteristic feature of French geology and geography, that all major cities are located in calcareous plains, while the mountains are low in calcareous deposits. A high urban mortality rate in the last century may also have been caused by high air pollution, poor microbiological and physical water quality and other factors. For categorizing water quality, Prof Louis-Claude Vincent used the so-called **"rH value"**, which describes the ratio between the redox potential and the pH value of a water.

The American physician *Dr Norman W. Walker* (1886 - 1985) always drank only distilled water and became almost 100 years old in the best state of health. However, it is always forgotten that he drank at least as much freshly squeezed fruit and vegetable juices from fresh, high-quality fruit and vegetables. Since fruit and vegetables are losing more and more of their value and vitamin content, this way of life is more and more difficult.

We can learn from Dr Walker that a diet of fresh, ripe fruits, well chewed or gently pressed into juice in a high-quality juicer, as completely and freshly as possible, is an effective and side-effect-free way to contribute to healthy ageing.

The rH value

The rH-value often used by Prof Vincent, for example, is widely only incompletely understood and applied, therefore, wrong conclusions are drawn from the work of Prof Vincent and his system of water assessment. The rH-value serves to assess whether a water has an oxidizing (i.e.

electron-robbing) or reducing (i.e. electron-adding, antioxidant) property by eliminating the impact of the acid-base effect of the pH-value on the redox properties of the water.

The calculation of the rH value is as follows:

$$rH = 2 \times pH + (2 \times eH) / 59.1$$

"eH" is the redox value measured with a standard hydrogen electrode as used in commercially available redox measuring instruments. This measured value must be corrected by a factor of 59.1 for the calculation.

The rH value is assessed as follows:

rH 0 - 9:	strongly reducing properties
rH 9 - 17:	predominantly slightly reducing
rH 17 - 25:	indifferent
rH 25 - 34:	predominantly weakly oxidizing
rH 34 - 42:	strongly oxidizing properties

If we calculate the rH value of an average alkaline ionised water with pH 9.5 and a redox value of -400 mV, we obtain:

$$rH = 2 \times pH\ 9.5 + (2 \times (-400\ mV)) / 59.1 = 5.5$$

If we calculate the rH value of an average acidic ionised water with pH 5.5 and a redox value of +600 mV, we obtain:

$$rH = 2 \times pH\ 5.5 + (2 \times (+600\ mV)) / 59.1 = 31.3$$

If we calculate the rH value of a strong catholyte with pH 13 and a redox value of -700 mV, we obtain:

$$rH = 2 \times pH\ 13 + (2 \times (-700\ mV)) / 59.1 = 2.3$$

If we calculate the rH value of a strong anolyte with pH 2 and a redox value of +1,100 mV, we obtain:

$$rH = 2 \times pH\ 2 + (2 \times (+1,100\ mV)) / 59.1 = 41.2$$

If we calculate the rH value of an average tap water with pH 7.5 and a redox value of +150 mV, we obtain:

$$rH = 2 \times pH\ 7.5 + (2 \times (+150\ mV)) / 59.1 = 20.1$$

If we calculate the rH value of an average reverse osmosis water with pH 6.5 and a redox value of +400 mV, we obtain:

$$rH = 2 \times pH\ 6.5 + (2 \times (+400\ mV)) / 59.1 = 265$$

What is the difference between alkaline ionised water and dissolved alkaline mineral powder?

The mechanisms of action of alkaline mineral powder dissolved in water and alkaline ionised water differ fundamentally. Alkaline mineral powders consist of mixtures of different salts of alkaline minerals and carbonic acid, citrate, sulphate, oxide or others, for example calcium carbonate (the carbonic acid salt of lime), potassium citrate, manganese sulphate or magnesium oxide. If these salts are dissolved in water, they react with it and "steal" an H^+ from the H_2O molecules, so that the minerals become positively charged mineral ions and the H_2O molecules become alkaline OH^- ions - a so-called **buffered solution** is formed. This buffered solution acts on the stomach acid by forming a salt between the alkaline mineral and the chloride of the hydrochloric acid, thus neutralizing it. This means that new gastric acid HCl can be formed from the sodium chloride NaCl dissolved in the blood. The resulting sodium surplus in the blood increases the blood buffer of sodium bicarbonate $NaHCO_3$ and thus the pH value of the blood. However, a higher blood pH value means that the oxygen can no longer detach so well from the haemoglobin – see chapter "Oxygen and carbon dioxide in respiration" – and that, despite sufficient oxygen in the blood, oxygen deficiency can occur in the tissue and in the cells. Furthermore, the removal of acid metabolic residues is also made more difficult. If alkaline mineral powders are taken regularly, there is the danger that the stomach will become accustomed to this neutralisation and will begin to form excessive stomach acid - this can result in heartburn and other stomach diseases.

Alkaline ionised water it is produced physically and not chemically, it is an **unbuffered solution** - it does not affect the production of gastric acid, as there is no alkaline mineral that can form a salt with the chloride of hydrochloric acid in the stomach and thus the hydrochloric acid cannot be neutralised. Alkaline ionised water is absorbed directly via the intestine and transferred to the connective tissue.

Is an alkaline diet better than taking alkaline mineral powders?

The increasing advertising for alkaline mineral powders suggests that it can permanently make up for a wrong diet with heavy acid content and wrong drinking with a lot of sugar and acids. Nevertheless, the intake of alkaline mineral powder only makes sense in order to neutralise acute (stomach) hyperacidity in the short term, but never in order to compensate for wrong lifestyles in the long term.

The reason is that alkaline mineral powder dissolved in water always forms ionised alkaline mineral ions (e.g. Na^+, Ca^{++}, Ka^+ etc.), regardless of whether the minerals were previously bound as citrate (sodium citrate, calcium citrate) or as carbonate (sodium carbonate, calcium carbonate etc.). Dissolved alkaline mineral ions cannot be properly absorbed by the intestinal mucosa, as both the intestinal mucosa and the alkaline dissolved minerals are positively charged and thus repel each other. Only a few fractions of the dissolved alkaline mineral ions can be absorbed in the large intestine.

It is different when alkaline mineral ions are embedded in larger plant structures, which can "dock" to the intestinal mucosa and be absorbed due to their at least partial negative charge.

So rather invest in healthy, organic vegetables, grown on soils with intact mineral status, than in alkaline mineral powders. If you need to supplement minerals - which is reasonable with a modern diet - make sure that you use a dietary supplement that is as natural as possible, gently processed, not heated over 30° C and based on organically grown plant concentrates.

Is alkaline ionised water an isotonic drink?

Isotonic drinks are touted as drinks that have the same properties (iso = equal, tonus = tension) as connective tissue fluid and lymph. Isotonicity is usually understood as the same **osmotic pressure** on both sides of a membrane, which means that isotonic liquid diffuses through the membrane only by mechanical pressure. Isotonic drinks have the same osmotic pressure as the body cells and are supposed to help athletes to replace minerals lost during sweating, as the osmotic pressure decreases due to mineral removal. In addition to minerals and vitamins, isotonic drinks contain fructose and glucose in order to quickly supply the body with energy.

However, in these considerations the **redox potential**, i.e. the electrical charge, is neglected. According to the principle of homeostasis, the body has to adapt everything it absorbs to its own environment. Since the connective tissue fluid and the blood have a negative redox potential between -5 and -60 mV, and the body cells can only absorb negatively charged water, but most beverages have a strongly positive redox potential, they are not isotonic from the point of view of the redox potential. Alkaline ionised water with its negative redox potential can therefore be labelled as an "isotonic" drink from the redox potential point of view.

Furthermore, the **water structure** is also neglected. All water in the body has small water clusters and a hexagonal water structure. Most drinks and tap water have a very large structure with large clusters. As alkaline ionised water has a very small and hexagonal cluster structure, it can also be labelled as an "isotonic" drink from the point of view of water structure.

What are the effects of alkaline and acid "water concentrates"?

Many brands of strong alkaline or acidic "water concentrates" are offered in health shops and different health effects are ascribed to them.

Catholyte, strong alkaline ionised water with pH-value up to pH 13, is produced by adding salt in special water ionisers. Depending on the type of salt (magnesium salt, sodium salt ...) and the way it is produced, catholyte has different tastes and different effects. Depending on the salt used, catholyte with pH values above approx. pH 10 taste soapy, bitter, salty or fishy.

To assess the quality of the catholyte, not only the composition and the pH value are important, but also and above all the redox potential of the diluted solution "ready to drink". If its redox potential has negative values, the catholyte has stored an excess of electrons able to survive the dilution with "normal" water. Then, the catholyte can have effects comparable to alkaline ionised water. In any case, the durability and stability of the high pH value and the negative redox potential must be considered.

Often special "information" and "informative effects" are ascribed to the catholyte. Since ionisation always involves breaking up and re-organizing the water structures, and a high salt concentration is also present, it may well be possible to permanently imprint certain oscillations and "information" in the catholyte. Here, however, critical caution is appropriate, since the production of simple catholyte is quite easy, it can be sold as an "informed" concentrate with high profit margins. On the other hand, "informing" may also require technically sophisticated equipment and processes, justifying relatively high prices. Therefore, "informational" effects should be tested subjectively and critically and neither be described as impossible nor simply believed.

Catholyte is offered for different purposes:

- As part of a **"de-acidification cure"**, catholyte should be taken either pure or diluted. Since catholyte is a partially buffered solution, it reacts with gastric acid and neutralizes it - "de-acidification cures" with catholyte should therefore only be carried out for a short time so that no habituation effect develops. They can be useful to accelerate the effectiveness at the beginning of drinking alkaline ionised water. In the long run, it certainly makes more sense to drink alkaline ionised water continuously than to regularly carry out a "de-acidification cure".

- As an **alternative to a water ioniser**, purchased catholyte does not make sense for cost reasons, since the running costs of the water ioniser are mainly due to the filter change - but a filter is also necessary for drinking tap water. Furthermore, adding catholyte cannot change the structure and size of the water clusters as good as a water ioniser.
- As a **short-term water ioniser substitute**, catholyte can, for example, serve to transform any water into alkaline ionised water during journeys.
- Catholyte can also be used to **refine dishes and drinks** - a drop of catholyte smoothens the taste of red wine or removes the acid flavour in coffee.
- "Informed" Catholyte can also serve as an "informational supplement" to alkaline ionised water.

Anolyte, strongly acidic ionised water, is used as an antibiotic, disinfectant and oxidizing agent for technical or medical applications. Since it is highly effective without building up resistance in microorganisms and is degraded residue-free, it is a useful alternative to many antibiotics and chemical disinfectants or oxidants. Since anolyte retains its oxidizing effect for a long time, it can be stored without losing its effect.

Therefore, using anolyte in farming, in animal breeding and also for disinfection in hospitals or – as in the recent corona virus pandemic – for large areas is a cheap, harmless and easily available alternative to the use of chemical disinfections and antibiotics.

What do urine and saliva pH values indicate?

It is often recommended to determine the body's acid-base balance by measuring the **pH value of the urine**. Measuring strips for measuring the urine pH value are sold in every pharmacy - but the user is left alone with the interpretation of the measuring results.

One has to bear in mind that the urine pH value only indicates what the body excretes, never the pH value of the body and the lymph itself. Therefore, an acidic urine pH value only means that the body excretes many acidic substances – this can, of course, indicate that the body is totally over-acidified, but it can also show that excretion works and that the body is able to get rid of the acids. If before measurement, acid-forming meals and beverages were consumed and/or acid excretion processes, diminishing old acid depots, were set in motion, an acidic urine pH value is a positive sign, indicating working body regulation functions. Acid excretion can be stimulated by fasting or changing the diet to a mineral-rich nutrition.

Therefore, permanently alkaline or only very weak acidic urine pH values are more critical: They show that the body does not excrete any acids via the urine. Of course, the reason may be that the body is very alkaline and the diet without acid-forming food and therefore no need for acid excretion exists, however it is more likely - particularly if health problems exist and the lifestyle is not extremely conscious, mineral rich and stress-free -, that the acid excretion via urine is blocked, causing endogenous hyperacidity. Anyone who thinks himself secure because of an alkaline urine pH value and considers further measures for de-acidification unnecessary, can then even harm himself.

If you want to read a usable statement from the urine pH value, you have to measure it a few times over the day and in relation to the meals and beverages consumed. Favourable and achievable with a reasonable and alkaline diet is a wide pH range, which means a strong acidic pH value - usually in the morning - and a higher, slightly alkaline pH value in the course of the day. If the pH range is small and the pH value fluctuates only slightly in the course of the day, problems are indicated, especially if the urine pH value is permanently slightly alkaline. A urine pH value that is permanently strongly acidic can indicate either a strong over-acidification with still functioning acid excretion, or a de-acidification process that is currently taking place, which can definitely be regarded as positive.

The **saliva pH value** approximately reflects the pH value of the body fluid. To measure it, it is important that you do not eat or drink anything except water at least two hours before measurement, and that you swallow your saliva several times before, so that really freshly formed saliva is measured. The pH-value of the fresh saliva should always be slightly alkaline. If it is acidic, it indicates acidic connective tissue or an acidic lymph and therefore, health problems.

An alkaline saliva is also essential for dental health, because caries is caused by the acidic excretion of caries bacteria. If the acids are neutralized by an alkaline saliva, they can cause less damage. The caries bacteria also develop primarily in an acidic environment, alkaline saliva inhibits their growth.

Serious illnesses such as diabetes or cancer are always accompanied by a low saliva pH value, therefore, chronically ill people usually have dental problems. Unfortunately, these connections are not yet statistically recorded, but confirmed by individual observations. They show that people suffering from cancer often have a saliva pH value below pH 6.

What can acidic ionised water and anolyte be used for?

With its very high redox potential, acidic oxide water and anolyte are **oxidizing agents** that rob bacteria and other microorganisms of electrons and thus oxidize and destroy them.

Depending on the mineralisation of the water, acidic ionised water from a normal water ioniser has a redox potential of over +600 mV. It can be used **to wash** hands, vegetables, fruit, kitchen utensils etc. and to disinfect utensils and small wounds. It is effective against skin diseases, insect bites and injuries.

Experiences of users show that it is also very well suited for **mouth disinfection**, for use in an oral irrigator, for **bathing (sweaty) feet**, for disinfection and cleaning of **small wounds** and **skin impurities** such as acne etc.

Anolyte, also called "super-oxidized water", which is produced with the help of salt in special water ionisers, has a redox potential of up to +1,100 mV at a pH of 1.5. Tests have shown that this water can even kill antibiotic-resistant bacterial strains and viruses.

Despite this strong disinfectant effect, acidic ionised water and the strongly acidic anolyte are completely safe, harmless and free of side effects. For example, the fish market in Tokyo is cleaned and disinfected with diluted anolyte, the Airport in Frankfurt, Germany, uses anolyte to clean and disinfect its tankers carrying water to the aircraft.

In Japan, acidic ionised water is successfully used for the treatment of **pressure sores** caused by prolonged lying, **open back**, **infected surgical wounds**, etc. There are also reports that it is used in combination with alkaline ionised water to treat **neonatal dermatitis**: The new-borns get alkaline ionised water for drinking and are washed several times a day with acidic ionised water. Thus, the neonatal dermatitis disappears without cortisone or other allopathic drugs and without side effects within a few weeks.

In Japan and Korea, anolyte is also used to treat **diabetic feet**. The feet are washed regularly with anolyte and the patient is given alkaline ionised water to drink.

It is also used in **agriculture**. In veterinary medicine, diluted anolyte is successfully used as an antibiotic substitute, e.g. for fattening pigs, as a disinfectant in the stable - for example for the udder treatment of dairy cows - and for general hygiene prevention. If it is nebulised in stables, the germ load decreases significantly. In arable and vegetable farming it is used to combat fungi and other plant diseases.

In Russia it is known that all hospitals are regularly disinfected with anolyte. The recent corona virus outbreak is fought in China with the widespread disinfection of streets, houses, shops, buses and so by spraying and nebulizing anolyte everywhere.

Acidic ionised water can also be used as water for cut flowers to disinfect, to prevent rotting and to slow down the flowering process. However, the flowers react differently, so that this must be checked in each individual case.

How can tap water be improved?

Tap water in so-called "civilized" societies is increasingly polluted by substances that originate from this very "civilization" and do not belong in the water. The waterworks have the thankless task of treating the local spring, ground or surface water contaminated with more and more undesirable substances in such a way that it meets the requirements of the national drinking water regulations – at a politically fixed price. In this respect, it is not surprising that the waterworks always have to compromise between the best possible purification and treatment and a price set by the politicians which has to be affordable for the citizens. Therefore, it is becoming increasingly important for health-conscious people to take the initiative themselves and to clean the few litres of water needed for drinking and preparing food in such a way that they not only comply with the official drinking water regulations, but also meet their own personal requirements to healthy water. Bottled water is not a sustainable alternative, not only for cost reasons, but also from the point of view of environmental protection, because of the immense burdens caused by transport and bottle production, cleaning and recycling.

In order to understand the pollution of raw water, the main sources of pollution are described here:

- **Pollution from contaminated sites and landfills**: Especially at old industrial sites, the soil is contaminated in many places by remains of former or existing commercial or industrial enterprises. From these polluted soils dioxins, polycyclic aromatic hydrocarbons (PAHs) and heavy metals can enter the groundwater and thus the raw water of the waterworks. Nowadays, these pollutants are mostly known and are usually treated in the best possible way - i.e. under cost-benefit aspects, with minimum costs.

- **Pollution from drug residues:** Allopathic chemical drugs are still at least partially effective after ingestion and excretion through the urine. Widely used drugs such as contraceptives, X-ray contrast agents, antibiotics and pain killers are often found in higher concentrations in raw water. More simply equipped waterworks that work without activated carbon filters can decompose complex chemical substances or hormones only to a very limited extent.

- **Pollution from (household) chemicals:** The exposure to these pollutants is increasing steadily. "Hygiene-conscious" households, commercial and industrial companies are using more and more chemical disinfectants and more sophisticated and complex chemicals for cleaning or material treatment. Their use is normally not regulated or restricted, therefore, the level of pollution through these chemicals in often unknown. These chemicals are also difficult to degrade.

- **Agricultural pollution:** Herbicides, pesticides and fungicides can be found almost everywhere in the world, spread also by air currents. In agricultural regions, besides herbicides such as glyphosate, a lot of liquid manure is spread, containing the residues of veterinary medicines - especially antibiotics. All these drugs eventually end up in the groundwater and then in the waterworks. To estimate how high the pollution level is at your place, you should ask your waterworks from which (groundwater) sources the raw water is taken. If it comes from an area with "critical" agriculture, such as conventional cultivation of wine, fruit or vegetables, or if many fields there are farmed conventionally and "treated" with liquid manure, fertilizers and pesticides, the probability of pollution is very high. If it comes from an area with forest, meadow orchards or pasture land, the pollution is likely to be lower. A "special case" are nitrates, which mainly originate from excessive fertilisation. Nitrates in themselves are only dangerous for babies under 3 weeks of age, as they have not yet developed an enzyme necessary for the degradation of nitrate – therefore, babies are not fed with spinach. In Germany, some new-borns died of cyanide poisoning due to a too high nitrate content of the water in the 1950th. Since then, nitrate has come into disrepute as a dangerous substance. Nitrate is actually harmless for adults, but it is often used as an "indicator" for pollution from conventional agriculture because it is usually accompanied by other agrochemicals and – different to chemical pollution – it is very easy to detect.

- **Pollution from the water pipeline network:** Even if a waterworks delivers well-purified water, it still has a long way to go before it comes out of your tap. Depending on the distance from the waterworks and the condition and age of the pipes, these can release traces of heavy metals or plastics. Nowadays, lead pipes can only be found in old buildings, but for example copper pipes soldered with lead solder are still possible sources of heavy metals. In countries without heavy tap water chlorination, a so-called "biofilm" forms in the pipe network, consisting of bacteria and other microorganisms. It increases if the water flows slowly because the pipes are oversized or because you live at the end of the pipe. This biofilm is stable and harmless as long as the water temperature is below 10° C, and it gets harmful only if the water stagnates in the pipe in higher temperatures, for example in the case of less used risers to a penthouse in an apartment building. Then harmful microorganisms such as legionella occur. In countries with heavy chlorination, the threat of microorganisms is eliminated, but therefore the chlorine itself is a harmful ingredient causing heavy oxidation problems. With heavy chlorinated water, harmful chloramines can occur.

- **Atmospheric pollution:** Air pollution increases the pollution of the soil and groundwater in the long term, even if the soil is still a very good filter and the microorganisms can decompose many air pollutants there.

- **Other pollutants** from car tyres abrasion, from lint from synthetic clothing, from the widespread rotting of plastic waste, from excreta from small animals living in the water pipes, etc...

Therefore, it is obvious that there is a "background presence" of pollutants in most of the tap water, caused by the "general civilization".

Basically, we can find different types of pollution in tap water. These pollutants have to be assessed and treated differently:

- **Organic chemical molecules** are difficult to analyse, as there are many tens of thousands of chemical compounds, and each substance must be specifically searched for. Therefore, in standard chemical water analysis, only a few frequently occurring chemical molecules are listed, a chemical analysis is always incomplete. For a comprehensive determination of organic chemical pollutants, water must be analysed in a well-equipped laboratory. This is expensive and the analysis is only valid for a short period of time, as chemical contamination can change at short notice and from day to day: For example, if a farmer spreads liquid manure on his field, the contamination can increase sharply the next day, but then disappears a few days after the next rain. An expensive and detailed chemical analysis is therefore not advisable, as it does not provide lasting safety. It is therefore important to filter all tap water used for drinking with a good activated carbon filter.

- **Heavy metals** are easier to analyse, heavy metal contamination is usually caused by the piping and is therefore permanent. It is therefore advisable to check the tap water for heavy metals. If heavy metals are really present, the cause can be searched for in order to carry out a remediation. Most heavy metals can be removed by so-called KDF filters.

- In countries with no or little tap water chlorination, the risk of **microbial contamination** occurs. It can be easily estimated: If water stagnates in the piping in a warm environment, there is a high risk of harmful bacteria developing. If the water is cool and flows regularly, there is hardly any danger. If microbial contamination is suspected, an analysis by an analysis laboratory can be carried out quickly and easily. Ultrafiltration elements or ceramic filter elements are suitable for the retention of microbial contaminants, also filters containing KDF are suitable for the prevention of increased risk of microbial contaminants. In the case of microbial contamination, all filters installed directly in the water pipe should be changed at least every six months or after a longer period of non-use, regardless of the amount of water flowing through, as bacteria can grow through filter media that are supposed to retain them. The bacteria growth curve begins to rise sharply after six months.

- Also, the increasing worldwide water contamination with **microplastics** makes it necessary to use appropriate filtration elements almost everywhere. For cost reasons, the waterworks cannot provide a solution. As with microbial loads, ceramic filters, ultrafiltration elements or fine activated carbon block filters are suitable for removing microplastics.

- Little is known about the fact that most pipelines also contain **isopods and other small animals** that feed on the bacterial film. Their excreta and dead animals are also found in tap water.

- **Nitrate** is a dissolved mineral, it cannot be filtered out by activated carbon filters, but can only be separated by a reverse osmosis system or exchanged for chloride ions in a nitrate ion exchanger. High nitrate levels are only critical for infants, but they are an "indicator" for agricultural contamination, which is much more difficult to measure and analyse.

- **Lime** is not a pollutant because it has no negative health effects. A high content of calcium in water is not dangerous, but only annoying. Lime can be removed by a reverse osmosis plant or by a lime ion exchanger, replacing it with sodium.

Unfortunately, dissolved minerals are often also considered as "pollutants". However, they are not pollutants, but natural substances contained in water, absorbed from the rock through which it flows. This consideration is particularly critical when an attempt is made to suggest a health hazard through high conductivity. However, a conductivity measurement only shows the total amount of substances dissolved in water - as a rule, at least 99.9% of all substances dissolved in water are natural minerals that have no negative health effects. Therefore, conductivity measurement is not suitable for the determination of pollutants.

Modern high-performance filters consist of various components, which should be optimally matched to each other and adapted to the water quality. These components are:

- **Activated carbon** is usually made of coconut shell or bamboo, as these materials are cheaply available and very fine-pored, but it can be made of all organic materials by charring and activation. Activated carbon has the property of adsorbing organic molecules, i.e. of attaching them to the activated carbon surface by electrochemical charge and permanently removing them from the water. This is done indiscriminately with all organic substances, so that activated carbon is recommended and useful as a standard filtration medium - even without analysis. The exact mechanism of adsorption has not yet been fully researched. In order to prevent bacterial contamination, activated carbon can be coated with silver or combined with KDF filter media.

  Several parameters are decisive for the filtration effect of an activated carbon filter:

  - **The pore size of activated carbon** and thus the contact surface between activated carbon and water is determined by the pore size of the raw material, but also by the quality of the treatment, i.e. whether all the finest pores are really "burnt free". Organic material, such as wood, has pores of various "size classes", from the coarse pores visible to the naked eye to the finest micro pores visible only under high-resolution microscopes. One gram of good activated carbon has an inner surface the size of a football pitch.

  - **The shape of the activated carbon**, i.e. whether it is loose granular activated carbon, pressed granular activated carbon or an activated carbon block with large or small pores, determines the intensity of the contact of the water with the activated carbon. A fine-pored activated carbon block reduces the water pressure, but the water molecules are pressed intensively against the activated carbon surface. Loose granular activated carbon, as it is used in simple household jug filters, leaves it more to chance whether a water molecule comes into contact with the floating activated carbon granules. In a thoroughly pressed granular activated carbon filter, the contact between water and activated carbon is intense, but the water can build "paths" through the activated carbon over time, on which it flows without much contact to the activated carbon surface. Generally, granular activated carbon also has the disadvantage that by shifting the granulate grains, the electrical charge and attraction can be disturbed in such a way that accumulated pollutants can be released again.

  - **The type and quality of activated carbon activation** also has an effect on the effectiveness of adsorption. Activated carbon is usually treated with oxidizing gas at 800 to 1,000°C or activated by chemical oxidation and thus obtains the adsorbing properties on organic molecules – the exact mechanism of which has not yet been fully deciphered. Activation can be reduced again by temperatures above 40°C - therefore activated carbon filters are only suitable for the filtration of cold and lukewarm water.

- **KDF filter media** (Kinetic Degradation Fluxion) consist of a high-purity copper-zinc alloy, to which cadmium, aluminium, iron, arsenic, lead, mercury and other heavy metals are attached to the surface by electrical attraction. Free chlorine, chloramines, hydrogen sulphide and other harmful compounds are broken down into harmless components and microorganisms such as fungi, bacteria, algae etc. are killed. The effect of KDF diminishes with high water hardness. However, KDF filters do not remove organic molecules and should be used together with activated carbon filters.

- **Ultrafiltration** usually consists of hollow filter threads closed at the water inlet side, open at the outlet side and having pores with a diameter between 2 and 100 nm. Water flows from the outside to the inside through the pores, so that bacteria, viruses, pigments, proteins, spores, microplastics and other microscopic solids etc. are removed, but dissolved minerals and salts are allowed to pass through. However, "normal" ultrafiltration media are not tested for manufacturing defects and can therefore not be used safely as a germ barrier to prevent bacterial contamination.

- **Bacteria barriers** are individually tested ultrafiltration elements which should be used for example before a reverse osmosis plant to prevent bacterial contamination, but also as an immediate relief if for example legionella are detected in the shower.

- **Calcium sulphate** granulate is used to bind free chlorine, raise the pH value and harden water poor in minerals. This is useful for reverse osmosis water, acidic water from granite rock or moor and swamp regions or surface water.

- **Ceramic elements** in a water filter have a pore sizes up to 0.2 µ and retain above all fine dusts and sediments. Due to the depth filtration effect they are also suitable for retaining microplastics, bacteria and other microorganisms. Since a ceramic membrane itself is a good growth medium for bacteria, it is often coated with silver. Ceramics are well suited as the first element in a multi-stage filter for water contaminated with sand or fine dust, as they can be mechanically cleaned of deposits and thus prevent clogging.

Decision guidance for the purchase of a water ioniser

Buying a water ioniser is an investment in your most important nutrient, drinking water, and in an appliance that you want to enjoy for a long time and to use with pleasure every day – it is therefore not worth making compromises in terms of quality, design or operating convenience of the appliance. Modern quality electric water ionisers from renowned Korean or Japanese manufacturers are sophisticated devices that have a long service life when used properly. On the other hand, there should be no costs for device features that are not useful and that have no effect on water quality or operating convenience – often too much technology is an additional unnecessary source of error or even breakdown. Therefore, we would like to address some aspects and criteria, which are important for the quality of the ionised water and the daily use, or where you can save money.

If you are planning to buy a water ioniser, the first thing you should decide is whether you prefer a mineral or an electric water ioniser. Both systems have advantages and disadvantages, but in addition to practical aspects, the decisive factor should also be a comparison of taste – which is often very individual, so that there is no clear "better" or "worse".

While mineral water ionisers are actually "extended water filters" and therefore – apart from regular filter changes and cleaning of the housing – require hardly any maintenance, electric water ionisers are complex electronic systems which have many features added by the time of their development and their performance is continuously increasing, even if the improvements are not really necessary for home use – of course at a corresponding price. Of course, some people also invest in cars going 250 km per hour or 150 mph, even if there is a national speed limit far below this figure. For this reason, some decision aids are listed here to give you criteria to decide which points are really relevant for daily home use and for you personally.

If you tend to use a mineral water ioniser, the following criteria should be complied with:

The **local water hardness**. The ionisation of the water is mainly the result of the reaction of the magnesium with the water. However, since the magnesium quickly coats itself with a layer of lime when the water has a high lime content and thus becomes ineffective, a water hardness above approx. 220 ppm $CaCO_3$ / 12°dH / 15°e / 22°fH is an exclusion criterion – unless you want to change the ionisation filter about every month.

Furthermore, units with **separate water and ionisation filters** are of course more flexible, as the water filter can be replaced every 6 months for hygienic reasons, and the ionisation filter can be replaced when the ionisation strength decreases.

	mineral direct flow water ioniser	electric direct flow water ioniser
Buying price	Lower	Higher
Replacement filter costs	Higher	Lower
Acidic ionised water	No	Yes
Maintenance effort	Lower	Higher, especially with hard water
Water flow	About 1 litre per minute	2 to 3 litres per minute
Amount of water	Max. 5 litres, then it needs a regeneration time of min. 5 minutes	unlimited
Amount of water per filter	Limited by the capacity of the bioceramic, filter change at least every six months or when the bioceramic is exhausted	Filter change every six months recommended
Maximum pH value	About pH 9 for 0.5 litres after the regeneration time	Up to pH 11
pH settings	No settings, regulation only by adjusting water flow speed	Mostly 3 to 4 steps
ORP value of alkaline water	Up to -400 mV	Up to -800 mV, depending on the source water
Connection	To water tap or mains	To water tap or mains and electricity
Water quality	Not recommended for hard water, works with RO water	Works also with hard water, but not with RO water
Process	Natural process by magnesium and bio-ceramics without electricity	Technical process by electricity, separation in alkaline and acidic ionised water

Table 8: System comparison between mineral and electric water ionisers

If you want to buy an electric water ioniser, you should consider the following criteria:

The maximum pH value is not the decisive criterion for a household water ioniser, as the optimum pH value for drinking is between pH 9 and pH 9.5. This value is reached by most devices for most water qualities. A maximum value of pH 11 may be an argument in terms of advertising, but it is just as useless in daily use as a maximum speed of a car of 180 mph. Furthermore, the achievable pH value always depends on the water quality, so that an advertised maximum pH value can be considerably lower for your tap water.

Likewise, **the size of the electrodes** is not decisive for the quality of the ionised water. Just like in a car engine, where a large displacement does not necessarily allow a conclusion to be drawn about its pulling power and force, the size of the electrode of an electric water ioniser is not decisive for the water quality, but rather the tuning of the control electronics, which "doses" the flow of electrons. It is also not decisive whether the electrodes are smooth, perforated or structured.

The type of platinum coating of the electrodes is also not really relevant. Electronic water ionisers from Asian production are usually equipped with titanium electrodes coated with platinum. Titanium is a material that is often used as an implant metal – be it for teeth or bones – because of its neutral properties and non-reactivity. Platinum is used as a catalyst. Catalysts are substances that intensify, accelerate or enable a chemical or physical reaction without themselves being involved. Just as platinum in the catalytic converter of your car accelerates the combustion of the nitrogen oxides NOx, the platinum coating on the electrode of an electric water ioniser accelerates and intensifies the formation of hydrogen H_2. The platinum coating is therefore not meant – as is often falsely claimed – to prevent the water from coming into contact with the titanium. Water ionisers from Russia, for example, often have untreated, pure titanium or even stainless-steel electrodes. There are two main methods for platinum coating of the electrodes: galvanic coating in an immersion bath with electrolysis – similar to an electroplating immersion bath used to galvanize the raw chassis of a car – or spray coating with a platinum spray similar to painting a car. Both methods certainly have some advantages and disadvantages, but the differences are limited and should not necessarily be decisive for a purchase decision.

Many water ionisers have a **display showing the pH value and OPR value** of the ionised water. However, as there are no maintenance-free sensors for measuring pH and ORP values, these displays are based on calculations only and are therefore unreliable. Comparisons of the displayed values with the values measured by a calibrated measuring instrument indicate deviations of up to 1.5 pH values and several 100-mV redox voltage. Instruments that display pH and redox values therefore feign an accuracy that is not available, so you can easily do without this display. If you want to have more accurate values, you have to measure both pH and redox values in the various setting levels at a defined flow rate and correct the displayed values accordingly.

Next to the common electric direct flow water ionisers, there are also so-called **pot water ionisers** in which the water is ionised by two electrodes in a container separated by a membrane. Here minerals and salts can be added and very high or low pH values can be achieved, i.e. **anolyte and catholyte** can be produced. To produce your daily drinking water, however, you need time and patience and, if possible, a drinking water filter, because a filter is not included with these devices.

Reasonable criteria for a purchase decision are:

A good activated carbon filter, preferably supplemented by a layer of **KDF filtration**, is a mandatory requirement if tap water is to be used for ionisation. Since tap water contains an increasing number of different residues of various chemicals from drugs, pesticides, herbicides, etc., but also heavy metals and other inorganic contaminants, these must be removed as completely as possible before electrical ionisation. If this does not happen, these chemicals are also ionised and thus chemically and physically altered in such a way that their activity becomes unpredictable. Depending on your tap water quality, you have to decide whether you need one or two filters – you always have to bear in mind that all filters should be replaced for hygienic reasons at least every 6 months or after a longer standstill without water flow – do not rely on the filter change indicator of the ioniser, since they do not know the contamination of your tap water and therefore cannot predict how many litres of water can be filtered. Changing the filter after 6 months is highly recommended because many studies show that bacterial growth increases exponentially after about 150 days. Therefore, it is recommended to always change the filter after a longer holiday if the water ioniser is not used during this time. It is therefore important to have a reliable filter from a trustworthy supplier who can guarantee that it will be available for the lifetime of the device.

Simple and reliable decalcification of the electrodes is also important. Due to the operating principle, the positively charged calcium ions attach themselves to the negatively charged electrode in the ionisation chamber and form a layer which impairs the flow of electrons and thus the functionality. For this reason, the polarization of the electrode must be regularly reversed so that the calcium ions adhering to the electrode are repelled and the formation of a lime layer is prevented. In simple devices, this is done by reversing the polarization for 30 to 60 seconds before each use, during which time acidic ionised water instead of alkaline ionised water comes out of the device. In more professional devices, this is done by using the two electrodes alternately as anode and cathode, which requires a complex control of the water flow. With these devices, alkaline ionised water is available immediately and without waiting time.

Independent of the decalcification of the electrodes, **regular decalcification and cleaning** of the device is also important. Depending on the water hardness and quality, this should be carried out quarterly to annually. A matured and practical cleaning concept is therefore a decisive argument for the durability and hygiene of a water ioniser. For cleaning, it has proven to be a good solution to pump vinegar or citric acid through the device with a pump or to use a special cleaning filter containing citric acid.

The type of water connection is decisive for the simple and convenient operation of the device. Simple devices are connected to the water faucet with a change-over water flow adaptor, but this has decisive disadvantages. Firstly, the change-over adaptor and the hose leading from it to the appliance restrict the freedom of movement of the faucet, and secondly, this connection is not possible with shower faucets without standardized threads. Furthermore, there is always the danger that hot water may accidentally flow into the ioniser. Even if hot water does not immediately damage the ioniser, activated carbon loses its cleaning activity through hot water and the filter must be replaced prematurely. It is therefore better to connect directly to the cold-water inlet under the sink and to use a regulating valve for the water flow directly on the appliance. Even more elegant, of course, are appliances that are located under the sink with an extra faucet mounted on the sink.

Last but not least, just as with the purchase of a car, **service** should also be a decisive factor in a purchasing decision: it should be ensured that spare parts and above all the specific replacement filters will still be available in a few years' time and that there is a workshop where your ioniser can be serviced and, if necessary, repaired.

Conclusion: The first question is the system decision between mineral and electrical water ionisers. For low lime tap water you have the best choice, because you can use both an electric and a mineral water ioniser without any problems. If your tap water contains a lot of lime, a reverse osmosis system with a mineral water ioniser might be an option.

If you want to buy an electric water ioniser: Just as there are no really bad cars nowadays, there are no really bad water ionisers anymore - at least if they are made by renowned manufacturers from Japan or Korea. In my opinion, it is still not advisable to buy Chinese products, which are often also sold as so-called "OEM products" with the name of an importer, as neither the quality nor the supply of spare parts can be guaranteed there. This does not mean, however, that there cannot be good products from China in the future. So, it makes sense to use similar criteria when deciding to buy a water ioniser as when buying a car: it should be a product from an experienced manufacturer, practical in use, suitable in design, and service and spare parts supply should be guaranteed.

Tips for handling electric water ionisers

An electric water ioniser from a renowned manufacturer is a durable device - provided that it is regularly serviced. To ensure that you can enjoy your water ioniser for a long time, you should follow some advice:

- The table-top **installation** of a simple electric water ioniser with a change-over water flow adaptor on a normal water tap is not witchcraft and can basically be done by yourself. An under-table installation is more complex and requires manual skill. Since the device is connected directly to the domestic water supply and is always under water pressure, we recommend installing a leakage protection. Ask your plumber if you are not sure whether you can do this yourself.

- If your water ioniser does not have automatic **electrode decalcification**, it is important that the electrodes are decalcified manually on a regular basis by reversing their polarization, i.e. you set "Acidic ionised water". Once "properly" calcified electrodes are very difficult to decalcify again, the lime can cause ionisation chambers to burst and thus destroy the unit. The harder your tap water is, i.e. the higher its lime content, the more frequently you should decalcify it. You can find out the hardness of your tap water from your waterworks. Here are recommendations without obligation:

  < 0.4 ppm $CaCO_3$ / 6 °e = soft: 30 seconds decalcification every 20 litres

  0.4 - 0.8 ppm $CaCO_3$ / 6 - 12 °e = medium: 60 seconds decalcification every 20 litres

  > 0.8 ppm $CaCO_3$ / 12 °e = hard: 60 seconds decalcification every 10 litres

- An electric water ioniser should be **decalcified and cleaned** as a whole at least every six months – preferably before changing the filter. This is done either by pumping a citric acid solution through the appliance in a circuit, or by special cleaning filters which are inserted into the filter housing and contain a cleaning granulate – usually also citric acid – which dissolves and decalcifies and cleans all water-carrying parts of the appliance.

- For hygienic reasons, the built-in activated carbon filter should be changed at least every **6 months**, as after 6 months bacteria begin to grow exponentially, which can lead to the entire appliance being contaminated – regardless of the amount of water used and the manufacturer's filter change recommendations. An earlier filter change may only be advisable if the water quality is very poor or the consumption is very high. It is not possible to determine the exact litre capacity of a filter, as the quality and load of the tap water would have to be known.

- Also, for hygienic reasons, you should remove the filter of your water ioniser and place it airtightly packed in the refrigerator (not in the freezer compartment!) if the device is not used for several days. Regular use is the best protection against bacteria, only when water is standing – e.g. in the filter – do bacteria find good growth conditions.

- We are often asked whether and how the ionised water can still be "energetically" optimized or "informed". Basically, it is possible and for those who believe it is worthwhile to do so, but there are so many different methods and procedures on the market – from quartz crystals in the glass carafe to energizing aids which cost more than the price of a water ioniser – that we cannot and do not want to make any recommendations. It is important – as these effects cannot be measured objectively – that you can test energizing aids with full refund rights on your own device in your home environment for a certain time.

- Glass bottles are best suited for storing and transporting the alkaline ionised water. Polycarbonate bottles are also suitable. Glass and polycarbonate are electrically neutral and do not affect the redox potential of the water, while other plastics and metals are electrically positively charged and immediately neutralise the reducing, antioxidant effect of the alkaline active water by drawing electrons from the water. In addition to their oxidative effect, PET bottles are also unacceptable because they can release chemical ingredients into the alkaline ionised water.

- Alkaline ionised water causes bottles and glasses to calcify faster. This is not a deficiency, but a natural process, as the dissolved calcium in the water is present in a so-called lime-carbonic acid balance, i.e. in tap water the calcium contained is neutralised by carbonic acid. During the ionisation process, the alkaline minerals and thus also the calcium are concentrated on the alkaline side, while the carbonic acid dissolved in the water is neutralised. Initially, the dissolved calcium is kept in suspension by the electrical charge of the alkaline ionised water – i.e. the redox potential – but as this charge gradually dissipates, the calcium precipitates and settles on the glass or bottle. It is best to clean calcified glasses and bottles with a citric acid solution.

Which drinking water treatment methods are available?

- In **reverse osmosis (R/O) plants**, the water is pressed through a membrane with a pore size of approx. 0.0001 µm or 0.1 nanometres, which allows only water molecules and dissolved gas to pass through, but forms a barrier for larger elements and molecules. The membranes are perforated with lasers and produced on an industrial scale – e.g. for seawater desalination. During production, ever larger holes are created, so that UO membranes are never bacteria-resistant and R/O water is never completely pure.

  Since the tap water from which reverse osmosis water is produced usually has a balance of lime and carbonic acid, and a reverse osmosis membrane filters out and rejects the lime, but allows carbonic acid and other dissolved (acidic) gases to pass through, reverse osmosis water contains these acidic gases and is almost always acidic – and usually the more acidic the more lime is contained in the original water.

  A direct ionisation of reverse osmosis water is not possible, because its electrical conductivity is too low. Before ionisation, salts or minerals must therefore be added to it to mineralize it

- **Distilled water** is very similar to reverse osmosis water, it is produced by evaporating and condensing (tap) water. Since all volatile substances with a boiling point below 100°C evaporate with the water, an activated carbon filter is added after the condensation, which adsorbs these volatile substances. Distilled water does not only need a lot of energy for its production, it is also very aggressive like reverse osmosis water, even if its pH-value is slightly higher. As with reverse osmosis water, direct ionisation of distilled water is not possible.

- **Ion exchangers** consist of electrically charged synthetic resin beads, the so-called "exchange resins", which, depending on their charge, attach and hold ions from the water. Calcium Ca^{++} is positively charged and requires a negatively charged resin, nitrate NO_3^- is negatively charged and requires a positively charged exchange resin. These exchange resins can be regenerated by concentrated saline solution $NaCl$, i.e. instead of Ca^{++} or NO_3^- molecules or atoms, sodium Na^+ or chlorine Cl^- accumulate on the beads, which are then replaced, i.e. exchanged, by calcium or nitrate again. Calcium is replaced by sodium, nitrate by chlorine.

  Ion exchangers are used to protect water pipes in highly calciferous or highly corrosive water or to remove lime and nitrates or other dissolved minerals.

  Water ionisers can be used without problems after an ion exchanger.

- **Can filters** also work according to this principle if they want to soften water. However, their synthetic resin beads cannot be regenerated; they are "loaded" with hydrogen which they release when they attach calcium ions. In these ion exchange filters working with hydrogen ions, the acidity of the water is increased.

- **"Sparkling" water** is made by adding carbonic acid to the water. Carbonic acid is carbon dioxide dissolved in water, a gas that humans and all mammals exhale, as it is an acidic waste product of combustion in the body's cells. "Sparkling" water is always acidic, this helps to prevent contamination by the bottling plant or by reusable bottles that have not been properly cleaned, but also simulates a non-existent freshness and liveliness of the water, which "disappoints" the body because the biological effect does not correspond to the sensation of taste. Apart from this, it is questionable whether it makes sense to force a gas back into the body through the water that the body has just exhaled. The "sparkling" of water is not a "treatment" in the sense of purification, but only the addition of a gas.

- **Levitated water** is produced by rotating water in a vertical pipe at a rapid rate. As it exits the top end, the water clusters are "torn apart" and reduced in size by the centrifugal force. Ionised water has equally small water clusters, but requires much less energy to produce. Levitation also does not remove any pollutants from the water - except dissolved gases.

- **Swirled water** is usually produced from tap water by tap attachments. The simplest way of swirling, however, is to connect two bottle openings, then the water can run from one bottle to the other with a swirl - swirling back and forth a few times can noticeably change the "consistency" of the water. Tap attachments swirl the water through specially arranged vortex chambers with the help of water pressure. There are also special electrically operated whirling devices available, which create whirls with different methods. Just as with levitation, swirling only changes the water structure and reduces the size of the water clusters, the chemical composition remains the same - except for possible outgassing of gaseous ingredients. Swirling ionised water is counterproductive, as hydrogen and electrons are "swirled out".

- **Oxygen water** is produced by adding oxygen. The oxygen molecule is surrounded by water molecules, but outgases easily. Oxygen water can increase the oxygen partial pressure pO_2 in the blood, but cannot compensate for the causes of too low pO_2, which is due to hyperacidity. Alkaline ionised water contains a lot of non-oxidizing oxygen due to the excess of OH^- ions.

- **Ozonized water** is produced by adding ozone (O_3). Ozone is a strong oxidizing agent and is used, for example, in public swimming pools to reduce the number of germs in the water. Ozonized water has a high redox potential and is very aggressive. Ozonized water is promoted with the increased content of oxygen – but the same applies here as for oxygen water, namely that oxygen in the water can at best increase the oxygen partial pressure, but never compensate for the causes of illnesses. It is questionable whether drinking such strongly oxidizing water makes biological sense.

- Systems for the production of water **sterilized with UV light** are also available, but this makes sense only if the tap water conditions are really bad and the tap water cannot be drunk directly. The ultraviolet radiation destroys microorganisms in the water, but leaves their "dead bodies" inside, which would be removed by small pore filters.

- **Hexagonal water** is a term coined by the Korean professor and water researcher *Mu Shik Jhon* for water with a hexagonal cluster structure. He found this water not only in the body as the water directly surrounding the cells and proteins, but also as glacier or fresh stream water in nature. Hexagonal water can technically be produced by swirling or ionisation - ionised water therefore is also hexagonal water.

- **Energized or vitalized water** is produced by various methods which can also be applied to water after ionisation – but often it is enough to take the glass of water in your hand and send it some good thoughts!
  - **Transmission of energy** (e.g. from spring water) influences the energy of the water molecules
  - **Minerals** (e.g. quartz) additionally transfer order structures
  - **Magnets** rotate the water molecules once around their own axis as they flow past, reducing and arranging cluster structures

How do I select a drinking water treatment system?

There are so many different methods of enhancing or treating tap water that it is often too much for the layman to decide which method to use.

A drinking water treatment plant can have three stages:

- The **purification**
- The **physical conditioning**
- The **enrichment**

The quality of the tap water at the site is the most important factor for the selection of the purification stage. If you have soft tap water, activated carbon filtration is sufficient. However, if you have tap water with a high lime content, you should consider a reverse osmosis system and further treatment.

Cleaning the drinking water from harmful substances is the mandatory part and compulsory before you start with the further enhancement of the water in terms of energy, physics and chemical substances.

In order to decide here, however, the **criteria** must first be established which should form the foundation of the decision. Since the effect on humans is the main focus of drinking water, these criteria are mainly the physical and chemical parameters that influence our health and have biological effects.

The biologically important parameters are:

- The **acid-base balance** (measured as pH): its importance has been explained in detail in the previous chapters. Good drinking water should therefore have a slightly alkaline pH value, i.e. between pH 8 and 9.

- The **redox potential** (measured in mV = millivolt or as rH-value): the significance of the electrical charge of water has also been explained in detail at previous chapters. Good drinking water should therefore have a negative redox potential - i.e. a redox potential with a negative sign - and a reducing (anti-oxidative) effect, i.e. an rH value below rH 17.

- The **cluster size**: The cluster size can only be measured with great effort, but it is important that good drinking water should have clusters as small as possible.

Indirectly affect the biological conditions:

- The **hydrogen content**: dissolved hydrogen is considered a new, selectively acting antioxidant. Alkaline ionised water contains dissolved hydrogen when it is fresh. The complex, comprehensive and diverse biological effects of hydrogen (as molecular hydrogen H_2, hydrogen gas) are currently being intensively researched worldwide.

- The **oxygen content**: Although the direct oxygen content is important for organisms living in water, it is of secondary importance for humans, since an increased content of oxygen gas (O_2) can increase the oxygen partial pressure in the blood in the short term, but does not have long-term effects. Oxygen in the form of an excess of OH^- ions - i.e. as an increased alkaline value - is biologically much more effective.

- **Conductivity** (measured in µS = Micro Siemens) or **resistance** (measured in Ω = Ohm): Pure H_2O does not conduct current, it has a high resistance and low conductivity, water with many dissolved minerals has a low resistance and high conductivity. Some "philosophies" claim that a high resistance is a sign for good water. However, since our body is an "electric" organism whose internal communication is based on the transmission of very fine electrical signals between cells, this assertion is not tenable. On the contrary, a high conductivity of water facilitates the transmission of signals. Also, water containing minerals has an ordered structure, whereas mineral-free water has no structure. Water with a certain amount of dissolved minerals - even if these cannot be absorbed directly - is therefore to be preferred to water poor in minerals. Conductivity and resistance are thus parameters that are only of indirect importance for the biological effect.

	Organic pollutants	Heavy metals	Nitrate	Chlorine	Lime	Dissolved gases
Can filter						
A. carbon granules						
A. carbon block						
Reverse osmosis						
Ion exchange						
Distillation						
KDF						
Reference	No reduction	Mini reduction	Light reduction	Partly reduction	Good filtration	

Table 9: Comparison of water filtration methods

	The pH value is …	The redox potential is …	The cluster size is …	The oxygen content is …	The hydrogen content is …
Magnet treatment	... unchanged	... unchanged	... slightly reduced	... unchanged	... unchanged
Boiling	... slightly increased by outgassing CO_2	... unchanged	... slightly reduced	... unchanged	... unchanged
Swirling	... slightly increased by outgassing CO_2	... unchanged	... strongly reduced	... slightly increased	... unchanged
Levitation	... slightly increased by outgassing CO_2	... unchanged	... strongly reduced	... slightly increased	... unchanged
Electric ionisation	... strongly increased	... strongly negative	... strongly reduced	... unchanged **	... slightly increased
Mineral ionisation*	... strongly increased	... strongly negative	... slightly reduced	... unchanged	... strongly increased
Electric hydrogen enrichment	... slightly increased	... strongly negative	... slightly reduced	... unchanged	... strongly increased
Reference	No change	Some change	Major change		

Table 10: Comparison of physical water treatment methods

* with elementary magnesium

** in the acidic ionised water, oxygen gas O_2 is formed, in the alkaline ionised water hydrogen gas H_2, but the total amount of oxygen or hydrogen is not changed, because it is balanced in the acidic ionised water by H_2OH^+ ions with low oxygen content, in the alkaline ionised water by OH^- ions with lower hydrogen content.